# Managing a
# Veterinary
# Practice

# Managing a Veterinary Practice

*Caroline Jevring*

BVetMed, MRCVS
Nordic Connection, Skyttevägen 9A,
133 36 Saltsjöbaden,
Sweden

**W.B. Saunders Company Ltd**
London • Philadelphia • Toronto • Sydney • Tokyo

W.B. Saunders        24–28 Oval Road,
Company Limited      London NW1 7DX, UK

The Curtis Center
Independence Square West
Philadelphia, PA 19106-3399, USA

55 Horner Avenue
Toronto, Ontario M8Z 4X6, Canada

Harcourt Brace & Company
(Australia) Pty Ltd
30–52 Smidmore Street
Marrickville, NSW 2204, Australia

Harcourt Brace Japan
Ichibancho Central Building,
22-1 Ichibancho
Chiyoda-ku, Tokyo 102, Japan

A catalogue record for this book is available from the
British Library

ISBN 0–7020–1987–9

This book is printed on acid-free paper

Typeset by LaserScript, Mitcham, Surrey
Printed and Bound in Great Britain by WBC Book Manufacturers,
Bridgend, Mid Galmorgan

# Contents

# Foreword

Practice management for veterinary surgeons has become an increasingly important subject. The business world has changed rapidly during the last five years due to a worldwide slow-down and increase in competition. Veterinary medicine has not been immune from these business world changes as growth of both the human and pet animal population have slowed, while the number of veterinary surgeons has increased. The current state is that more and more veterinary surgeons are chasing fewer and fewer clients.

The practice of veterinary medicine must be refocused from our past habits of just treating disease to a future position of offering complete preventative health programmes. A new vision of professional service will be needed to meet the needs of the new, better educated consumer.

The most successful veterinary medical practices of the future will devote as much effort into 'how' services are delivered as they spend on the quality of the services delivered. The important issues of communication, leadership, motivation, client development, and business management will be required to be mastered and practised alongside professional knowledge.

Our future practice success depends on our ability to understand and manage change. Change must be perceived as opportunity and not as a threat. This text offers insight into how to understand and manage change and how to improve the delivery of services to meet the client and patient needs of the future.

Excellence in the quality and delivery of professional services will provide our clients, patients and the profession with the level of care that we are dedicated to perform. Veterinary surgeons in all locations in the world are focusing on improving quality and delivery of services through commitment to continual improvement. It has been my good fortune to be able to work with and share information about veterinary practice management in many countries in the world. I have been richly blessed by my association with colleagues such as the author of this text, Caroline Jevring, and her husband Jan Jevring.

This book was written to provide current, positive and professional information about improving our practices to better meet the needs of our patients and clients.

*Dennis M. McCurnin*, DVM
*Diplomate, ACVS*
*Baton Rouge, Louisiana*
*USA*

# Introduction

*Good practice management is good veterinary medicine*
Lord Soulsby, June,1994

The world recession forced the veterinary profession up against the wall. Practitioners panicked, some practices went bankrupt – but some not only survived the recession, they flourished. Why? Because they actively and positively responded to their changing environment.

Although the veterinary profession contains many dedicated and hard-working members, as a whole I believe it is in danger of being too conservative and resistant to new ideas for its own good. The frustration this generates, especially amongst the younger veterinarians, is reflected in the number that leave practice, and even leave the profession altogether. Much of the resistance comes from not knowing *how to respond to change*. This book is my attempt to help veterinarians in practice face change boldly and confidently.

If there is one word which could summarize many of the concepts in the book it would be *planning*. Planning is an essential component for success in most areas of practice, from planning annual financial performance targets to planning your marketing. In fact, you can plan your own success by calculating what you want to achieve, working out how you can achieve it, setting yourself a time-frame in which to achieve it – and then going for it!

Veterinary practices are small businesses. To be successful they need to well managed. This has traditionally been one of the various roles of the practice principal. However, he or she may not be the best person to do it. What are the options? If principals employ practice managers will this free them to practice better standards of medical and preventive care in the practice?

This book focuses on some of the key management issues practitioners need to know about such as clarifying what the practice stands for, what their role as principal/leader/manager/owner/clinical veterinarian in the practice really means, how to develop and empower staff, and how to improve staff and client relations through better communication skills to create a happier practice with more satisfied clients. It contains many basic business management principles although it is not a complete management manual; for example, there is very little on practice finances.

I hope this book will be of use to you, or, at the very least, be thought-provoking!

*Caroline Jevring, BVetMed, MRCVS*

# Acknowledgements

My most grateful thanks go to family and friends who have helped and advised me, especially Nils Friske, senior business management consultant; my parents, Sally and Bernard Stonehouse; my brother, Paul Stonehouse; and my long-suffering and patient husband, Jan Jevring. A very special thank you goes to Dennis McCurnin whose lectures and enthusiasm for the subject of practice management have been my source of inspiration.

## Dedication

*For my sister Ann, with love. Without your encouragement and advice this book would never have been written.*

# 1 Creating the Will for Change

*The assumptions on which the organization has been built no longer fit reality. These are the assumptions that shape any organization's behaviour, dictate its decisions about what to do and what not to do, and define what the organization considers meaningful results ... (The organization's) ... theory of business no longer works.*

Peter Drucker, Senior Management Consultant

THE one consistent feature of today's business environment is change. As change, by its very nature, is continuous, then the successful business must be flexible and adaptable – the responsive organization.

The business of veterinary practice is no less exempt than any other from the challenges of change. In recent years, these have ranged from a world recession and new European Union legislation, to the demands of more knowledgeable clients and altered expectations of new graduates. Indeed, one of the greatest challenges has been to recognize that the veterinary profession is a service profession, serving the needs of the animal owner and their animals.

The successful practice must therefore be a responsive practice: *the practice that makes every effort to sense, serve and satisfy the needs and wants of its clients within the constraints of the ethical standards of the veterinary profession, and the financial resources of the practice.*

## The impact of change

If not properly managed, change can decrease morale, motivation and commitment within an organization and create conditions of conflict. Resistance to change is natural. It arises because of:

- *Preference for stability.* People seek to maintain their equilibrium.
- *Habit.* Habits, once established, provide comfort and satisfaction.
- *Conformity.* For many people anything that diverges from the accepted norm in their environment is disruptive and disturbing.
- *Perceived threat to own interests.* People focus on their own best interests and think that any change must be for the worse. Often, they only take the short-term view of the immediate difficulties to be overcome.
- *Misunderstanding.* People may not understand the implications of change and believe it will cost them much more than they will gain.
- *Fear of the unknown.* Ambiguities in goals, roles and the methods of achieving the new goals and measuring the response create fear and uncertainty.

Change is a threat to familiar patterns of behaviour as well as to security, status and financial rewards.

## ■■■ Change and the veterinary profession

Veterinarians are as wary of change as anyone. But change need not be frightening if you know how to approach it. I have broadly divided the challenges facing the profession into three areas; external ('world') factors, external (client) factors, and internal factors (see Figs 1.1 and 1.2). The external ('world') factors are things such as the world recession or

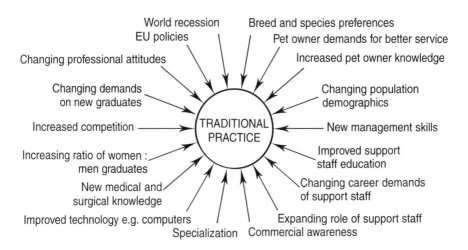

**Fig. 1.1** *The need for change: some of the factors influencing traditional practice.*

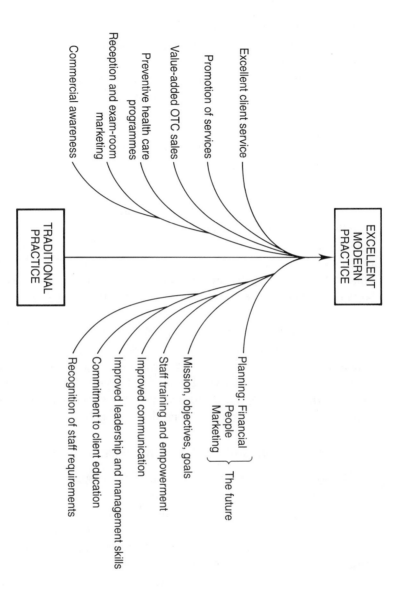

**Fig. 1.2** *Some of the management factors needed to convert the traditional practice to the excellent modern practice. OTC, over the counter*

advances in general technology over which the profession has very little or no influence. External (client) factors include the changing demands clients make on the profession, and represent the major area of opportunity and progress for the profession through education and marketing. The internal factors reflect the attitude and feelings within the profession itself, and although they are completely under the control of the profession, they are often the major source of limitations within the profession.

# External ('world') factors

## World recession

The world recession, from which many countries are emerging, has had a significant effect on all businesses, not least veterinary practice. Practices which in the late 1980s were expanding confidently, opening new branches and taking on new staff, were forced, in the 1990s, to pull in their horns as client numbers dropped and client spending fell. Once-full waiting-rooms were nearly empty, clients were more reluctant to choose complicated (and therefore more expensive) treatment options, and practice incomes dropped significantly. Veterinarians faced a dilemma: should they sit and wait for clients to come in as they had always done, or should they review their practice policies and go out to their clients with improved programmes of health care and better service? Those practices which saw the recession as an exciting challenge and an opportunity for development not only survived but did well. How did your practice respond?

## EU and national veterinary associations

Throughout the EU, practice standards, drug dispensing legislation and standards of animal care are under review as well as animal transport and movement regulations, and slaughter legislation. On a smaller scale, national veterinary associations such as the British and American veterinary Association are constantly updating and revising veterinary legislation. What needs to change in your practice to fulfil the new requirements? Who of your staff needs extra information or training?

## Modern technology: computers

Computers are an essential modern business tool, and yet many practices are still not computerized. Computers are an invaluable aid for managing the practice accounts, payroll analysis, stock control and costings, clinical records, word processing, reception control, preventive health pro-grammes, marketing and much more besides. Although this book does not dwell in depth on the choice of computer or all the tasks that a computer can perform in practice, the importance of the computer in a modern practice is highlighted throughout.

### The value of the pet industry

The pet industry is Big Business. With over 50% of the British population owning pets, many of these as multiple pet households, the British pet industry was valued at £2.5 billion in 1993. Veterinary practice is part of that business. By not only treating sick animals but providing preventive screening and health care services such as obesity, senior, behaviour and dental programmes for healthy animals, veterinary practitioners expand their share of it. Are you getting your fair share?

## External (client) factors

### Serving the client

Veterinary practice is a service industry, committed to serving the needs of pet owners and their pets. The modern veterinary surgeon must satisfy demands for good service from increasingly better informed and discrimi-nating pet-owners, rather than relying on expertise in medicine and surgery to automatically ensure a successful practice.

### Human–animal bond

In the last 50 years the strength and value of the human–animal bond has been increasingly recognized. In most families, the companion animal is regarded as a family member. Informed owners want loving care for their pet, and seek to improve the health and life-expectancy of their friend through health-screening programmes.

Pets serve many functions. A dog, for instance, can be kept as a guard, a loving companion, a pet for the children, an incentive to exercise, a child/ family substitute, independence (for a blind person, say) and much more. Pets have been shown to improve human health and longevity, and serve a unique function in helping handicapped and institutionalized people.

Not only can animals have a huge personal value to their owners, but they may be very valuable in their own right for breeding, showing and racing. Owners of these animals also want to keep them in top condition.

How can practices respond to the needs of these different categories of owners? Could preventive health care programmes be part of the answer?

### Pet preferences

Pet species preferences have altered as more single-person households and joint-income families make money and time scarce commodities. There is a slow trend towards exotic pets such as birds, snakes and chinchillas, but the most marked trend is in the increasing ratio of cats to dogs.

Cats are probably the pet of the future. Many large cities have feline clinics that cater to the special demands of the cat owner. Incorporating a feline-only section in your veterinary clinic shows that you recognize that the cat is not just a small dog, but that, like its owner, has different and special needs.

### Changing social trends

Society has altered from a predominantly rural to a predominantly urban society. Fewer people are brought up with or have regular contact with animals (wild or domestic) and, as a result, have little or no idea of animal care or husbandry. The veterinarian is the best qualified person to help them choose an appropriate pet for their lifestyle, and to advise on pet behaviour, nutrition, housing, breeding, and general care, but how many companion animal practices promote this 'animal husbandry' aspect of their practice?

### Increased choice

Most people own cars these days which means travel to the veterinarian of their choice is easier and they are no longer bound to the nearest practice. Clients choose their practices based on convenience of locality, cost of the services, the perceived value of the services, and the quality of client service they receive. In many areas, the standard of client service has become the major differentiating factor in determining which practice they will visit. How do you influence your clients' choice?

## Internal factors

### Traditional practice image

For many pet owners, a traditional image of practice persists: the dedicated, caring veterinarian who works selflessly all day and night fixing sick and injured pets, working miracles because 'animals can't talk, can they?'.

Veterinarians know that modern practice simply is not like that. But how many take the time to explain this to their clients? Yes, practice is peopled by dedicated caring professionals who often do work seeming miracles, but this is because modern practice is so well equipped, and professional work standards so high. How many veterinarians take the time to show clients around the practice premises and show them what they do, show them the equipment and facilities in the practice, the preventive health care programmes, the value of the trained staff, the level of expertise at which the practice works? By perpetuating the myth of practice, veterinarians are performing a grave disservice for themselves because they reduce and limit the expectations of their clients.

### Changing professional attitudes

Young professionals have a different set of professional and personal values from their predecessors. Enthusiastic, creative and energetic, many are crushed into cynical apathy only a few years out of university because the profession refuses to recognize their needs. For many graduates, becoming a veterinary surgeon is no longer a vocation, it is a job. Twenty-four hour dedication 365 days of the year is not acceptable; young veterinarians want quality time off to pursue family and leisure activities.

Increased mobility offers the modern graduate a much greater chance of trying out a variety of practices in different parts of the country, or even abroad, and so develop a wider range of experiences. If and when they do settle in a practice, many veterinarians do not then want the heavy financial and emotional commitment of a full business partnership; they want instead to retain the freedom to make choices, especially if their spouse also has career decisions to make.

How do you accommodate the needs of young professionals and support staff in your practice?

### Women in the profession

Women have accounted for well over half of new veterinary graduates for the past 5 years, yet many women still face sexual discrimination from male colleagues and clients. Young women graduates are paid on average nearly 10% less than their male colleagues (Hill, 1993), and there are far fewer women practice principals and specialists.

By the year 2000, women will probably form the majority of the veterinary workforce. A caring profession demanding intelligence and dedication, it is one to which women are well suited. However, the profession has not yet come to terms with developing policies which will suit the career needs of women while balancing their needs for flexible time to care for a family. How adaptable and supportive is your practice to the needs of its female members?

## Stress and stress management

Stress arises from an inability to balance high professional standards with personal fulfilment. It can lead to alcoholism, drug abuse, 'burnout' and suicide, and is an increasingly serious problem among members of all the caring professions.

Members of the veterinary profession are especially prone to stress and this is reflected in it having the highest suicide rate of all the professions. Stress starts early as the recent SPVS young graduates survey showed: 15.6% of those who answered said they were discontented and more women graduates were discontented than men. Elkins and Elkins (1987) in their survey of professional 'burnout' amongst American veterinarians, found that those in the 10–14 years-in-practice group had significantly higher scores for predisposition to 'burnout' than other groups.

Active steps to help veterinarians are already being taken in Britain with the Veterinary Helpline, a telephone helpline manned by a small cadre of voluntary workers (themselves veterinarians or spouses of veterinarians) who can act as 'befrienders' rather than counsellors to veterinarians with personal or business problems. Supported by the British Veterinary Association and the Royal College of Veterinary Surgeons, it has already helped a number of distressed or worried veterinarians. But what more can be done – perhaps even at pre-university entrance and student level – to help members of the veterinary profession to prevent further loss through disillusionment, despair and untimely death?

## Veterinary knowledge

Twenty years ago, the doubling rate of knowledge was measured in years; today it is only a few months. The rapid increase in the volume of veterinary knowledge makes specialization at a species and even a systems level essential. The RCVS Guide to Professional Conduct, 1993, clearly states that ' . . . *it is an ethical obligation on all veterinarians to ensure* . . .

   (b)   That after graduation they participate in a formal programme of continuing professional development.

(c)  That in the event of a major change in professional activity or after a career break, they undertake a period of further training and updating of skills sufficient to provide a full professional service'. (Section 1.2 Post graduation responsibilities, pp.10, 11.)

Continuing professional development (CPD) maintains professional expertise and is an essential part of excellent client service. Clients trust their veterinarian to provide the best possible care for their pet. Practices can encourage continuing professional development by paying for members to attend meetings, lectures and conferences as well as allowing time for further study towards specialist certification – but how many do?

### Competition

> *Most people . . . see life as a finite pie: if somebody gets a big piece of the pie then it means less for everybody else . . . People with a scarcity mentality have a hard time sharing recognition, credit, power or profit. They also have a tough time being genuinely happy . . .*
> Stephen Covey, Covey Leadership Centre

There are more veterinarians and veterinary practices than ever before. Additional competition comes also from other animal care 'experts' such as breeders and pet-shop owners.

Veterinarians are often frightened of what they see as competition because they have a scarcity mentality: they believe there isn't enough 'pie' to go around. Many fight colleagues by underpricing services, against the pet shop by slashing profit margins, and against the breeder by categorizing them as ill-informed and therefore dangerous.'Pies' are usually bigger than they seem, and competition can be converted to opportunity – the opportunity to work co-operatively, and give everyone a nice big piece.

How can you convert local competition to an opportunity to develop your business and serve your clients better?

## The way forward: creating the responsive practice

There is interest within the veterinary profession to respond to the challenges of change, but thinking, in general, is muddled. Practices commonly make only superficial changes to the way they do things – for example, they put up a few posters in the reception area, and repaint the sign outside and call this 'marketing'; or they write a business plan at the beginning of the year which is then disregarded for the rest of the year and call this 'business management'. To create the responsive practice requires deep-seated changes in attitude, understanding and actions. This new way of thinking is called a paradigm.

A paradigm is a viewpoint, a way of perceiving things. It has been likened to a pair of glasses, and just as changing your glasses gives you a different and often clearer view of the world, so changing your paradigm gives you a clearer view of the world. A paradigm change has to come from the inside, from looking at the way *you* think and behave and modifying that *before* you can start making changes in the practice. It is not easy – but the results are immensely rewarding and satisfying.

This book aims to create some new paradigms for you. It will show you not simply how to face change, but how to create the lust for change in your practice through good management, which will result in a successful, responsive practice. The following section summarizes the major issues presented in each chapter. The principles of responding to change are the same for every type of practice and although the examples given are primarily drawn from my own experiences with companion animal practices, they serve equally well to illustrate the situation in farm, equine and other practices.

## Overcoming resistance to change

Whilst people often take an antagonistic or negative attitude to change, it is also true that the desire for new experience underlies much of human behaviour. Bearing this in mind, you can take the first step towards creating the responsive practice by creating the right environment for change:

- Avoid *imposing* changes and new ideas on your staff – let them recognize and develop them themselves.
- Wholeheartedly support responsiveness and a desire to try new things.
- Ensure that changes create a better practice.
- Ensure that the changes are stimulating and interesting for staff.
- Involve staff in the change process.
- Gain agreement from all in the practice about the importance and value of changes.
- Ensure staff do not feel threatened by the changes.
- Adopt patience and tolerance.
- Allow plenty of constructive discussion so that there is complete understanding of new proposals.

People support what they help create. Commitment to change and to creating the responsive practice will be greater if those affected are allowed to participate as fully as possible in planning and implementing it. The aim of the practice leader is for the staff to feel they 'own' the change: it is something they want and are glad to live with.

## ■■■ Defining veterinary practice as a business (Chapter 2)

A veterinary practice is a small business. A business is an organized approach to a market. Veterinarians are not business people by nature or training but by learning to plan, organize and focus business efforts, adapting and modifying what the practice has now to the changing needs of the market, business success can be assured.

The one word which best sums how to develop the responsive practice is *planning*. Planning is the key to business success and is essential to manage change. Planning consists of five stages:

- defining a goal;
- working out how to achieve the goal;
- ensuring full understanding and collaboration of all involved in achieving the goal;
- monitoring performance and modifying the methods accordingly;
- rewarding success.

A business plan starts with defining a practice mission which crystallizes, in a few short sentences, what the practice is, and what it stands for.

The next stage of management is planning the development of the three major areas of the practice in relation to the mission. These are:

- the people plan;
- the marketing plan;
- the financial plan.

It is beyond the scope of this book to discuss how to formulate a financial plan, although advice is given on the controversial issue of fee-setting in Appendix 1. The people plan and the marketing plan are discussed in Chapters 6, 7 and 8.

# ■■■ Leadership and management (Chapter 3)

*The management of a veterinary practice is as much a specialized skill as are making a diagnosis, performing surgery, or evaluating a radiograph.*
Dennis McCurnin, Veterinary Practice Management Consultant, 1988

Strong leadership is a hallmark of a successful practice. A leader should have the vision that drives the practice forward· ɩ manager facilitates that vision by creating the atmosphere in which it can be achieved. In veterinary practice, the leader and manager are often the same person. This can create problems for the owner–veterinarian trying to juggle leadership with management with being a veterinarian.

Practice management is not about throwing away all the old values and concepts and bringing in new, trendy ones; it is about applying structure and systems to the old ideas so that they are more effective. Hiring a good practice manager can significantly reduce some of the stresses of running large, busy practices.

# ■■■ Improving communication (Chapters 4, 5)

Happy staff make happy clients: happy clients provide business. Good communication creates trust which is the cornerstone of successful business and is an essential part of client service.

Communication is a very complex skill involving the five senses. Because it is so complex, breakdowns in communication arise frequently and are a very significant source of problems such as job dissatisfaction, inter-staff tensions and low staff productivity. Poor communication also creates a lack of co-operation from clients, and can even cause clients to leave a practice. How can you improve communication in your practice?

# ■■■ Empowering your people (Chapters 6, 7)

Having excellent staff starts with hiring the right people, then coaching them to greater effectiveness. A good leader can convert people to a team through motivation,delegation and empowerment skills as well as constant performance assessment.

## ■■■ Quality client service (Chapter 8)

Clients cannot judge a practice by the standard of medical or surgical care they receive, but they can and do judge the level of service. The responsive practice requires people-orientated staff who provide what its clients want – excellence in service. To achieve excellence in service requires total commitment by the whole practice to the concepts of client service.

## ■■■ The role of preventive health care (Chapter 9)

Most of the dangerous infectious diseases are now controlled, and companion animals are living longer due to vaccination, parasite control and better nutrition. Pet owners want their pets to live healthier, fuller lives so practices need to change from providing reactive service to proactice service – that is, from treating disease to disease prevention. A very important but undervalued service to clients and their pets is preventive health care (PHC).

Effective PHC programmes are aimed at educating clients to make informed decisions about their pet's health. They require careful planning, staff education and a long-term outlook on what they hope to achieve. Many PHC programmes can be run predominantly by trained support staff, and contribute significantly to practice income.

## ■■■ The value of retailing in practice (Chapter 10)

The American trend towards 'one stop shopping' has encouraged the client convenience concept of providing all animal care services under one roof. Some of the large pet-superstore chains are already offering these services by having a veterinary practice within the shop. The veterinary profession, however, is still fairly resistant to the idea of retailing, regarding it as inapproriate and unprofessional in a clinic or hospital setting.

Professional retailing, properly organized, provides value-added service to clients, improves pet health by ensuring clients use veterinary-recommended products and simultaneously creates a vigorous profit centre for the practice.

## ■■■ Practice marketing (Chapter 11)

The aim of marketing is to establish your practice in the minds of your clients as being unique and different from all the other practices. Marketing is much more than simply advertising. It is the communication of the value of professional goods and services to clients. It is performed both internally and externally. Correctly used, it is a powerful method to develop your client base and increase profitability.

## ■■■ Looking to the future (Chapter 12)

The final chapter looks to the future. Conservative by nature, many changes are needed in attitude and behaviour within the profession for it to survive and flourish.

## ■■■ Summary ■■■■■■■■

1　Change is constant and continuous.

2　To have a successful practice veterinarians need to review their own paradigms and create the responsive practice.

3　Practice management, the skilful use of resources in a practice to create an organized approach to a specific market, is an essential component of the responsive practice.

# 2 Business or Bust?

*We cannot direct the wind but we can adjust the sails.*

Anon

A BUSINESS is an organized approach to a specific market. A successful business is one that changes and adapts to the changing needs of its market. The business of veterinary practice is serving animal owners through commitment to the health and welfare of their animals. The market for veterinary practice is animal owners, and as with all markets, their needs are constantly altering. The responsive practice is able to continually and enthusiastically metamorphose to serve these changing needs.

Britain is still suffering the after-effects of the world economic recession. During that recession some practices collapsed; the majority more or less survived. But a handful – those responsive practices that changed to meet a changing world – thrived and expanded.

I have visited many hundreds of veterinary practices and can identify eight features that characterize these responsive practices:

- *An overriding awareness of the needs and requirements of clients.* Practices use techniques such as active listening and client questionnaires to keep in close touch with the needs of their clients.
- *A predisposition towards action.* These practices actively seek business opportunities.
- *An independent attitude coupled with a willingness to be creative and imaginative:* an entrepreneurial and novel approach to practice development exists in these practices.
- *Simultaneously flexible and adaptable.* Top practices move and change with the times, and they plan carefully for the future, but the plans are not written in tablets of stone: they can be quickly adapted, modified or even discarded to suit new market forces.
- *An applied approach motivated by strong values.* These practices are driven by values such as professional and personal integrity, honesty and a desire to improve the health of animals in their care.

- *Productivity through people.* These practices recognize that their most valuable asset is their people and everyone in the practice is empowered to perform to the best of their ability.
- *Stick with the business they know.* Top practices establish expertise and stick to it.
- *Simple staff structure with minimum staff.* The top practices hone their staff to a minimum, and have a simple hierachical system. For example, each partner takes responsibility for a group of staff to inform them about decisions in the practice; or, a head nurse is responsible for each section of a hospital.

## ■■■ Chronic problems that apply to veterinary practices

So, why aren't more practices more successful? I believe it is a complex combination of issues which includes lack of interest, feelings of low self-esteem, and lack of leadership and management skills (summarized in Table 2.1). Too many veterinarians open their own practices without a truly clear idea of what they want to achieve with their practice.

As students, veterinarians are given little self-value; they therefore have difficulty in setting a value on themselves and their services when they qualify. They are not taught specific business skills at any stage of their career and they seldom have the chance to see good business principles in action. Assistants are not paid salaries according to their real worth; their

**Table 2.1** *Summary of poor management issues that affect practice productivity*

- Lack of vision and purpose
- Overdependence on specific individuals – often the practice principal(s)
- Poor leadership
- Low trust between the leader and staff
- Lack of integrity
- Failure to establish and/or communicate the practice's goals both within the practice and to the clients
- Lack of financial planning and review
- Lack of management systems
- Poor market segmentation and /or strategy
- Increasing competition and a lack of market knowledge
- Inadequate capitalization
- No standardized quality programme
- Concentration on the technical rather than the strategic work in hand

salary does not usually directly reflect the income they generate, so they do not relate proper charging with income generated. Practice principals are often technically very competent but are not very effective business managers, so much business in practice is inefficient and run by crisis management. Furthermore, veterinarians are traditionally taught to work reactively rather than proactively – that is, wait for clients to come to them rather than seeking to generate work. Finally, veterinarians are only just beginning to accept that they should regard their practices as real business concerns. As a result, practices lack goals, objectives and missions.

Most veterinary practices seldom fulfil more than a fraction of their business potential so how can these problems be overcome to create the responsive practice?

## ■■■■ Planning for success

Successful business depends on planning. Planning how to run your practice gives you control over your and the practice's destiny. There are three major, overlapping areas that require planning in practice (see Fig. 2.1 with some of the factors that need to be considered):

- financial;
- people (Chapters 5 and 6);
- marketing (Chapter 11).

Planning puts structure and systems to the current ideas you have in the practice; it is not necessarily bringing in lots of new ideas. Planning can be both short- and long-term; for example, what is the situation with your practice market now? In 2 years? In 5 years? By finding time to study trends and patterns for small business in general, to talk to friends in other businesses and members of other professions, and to read about business trends you can relate this information to your practice and its future. Invite management consultants to your practice or simply talk with colleagues in your practice so that you can formulate effective plans for the development and success of your practice.

## ■■■■ The practice life-cycle: where are you now?

Businesses are not static – they evolve with time. Maister (1986) has defined a practice life-cycle for professional service firms. He suggests that

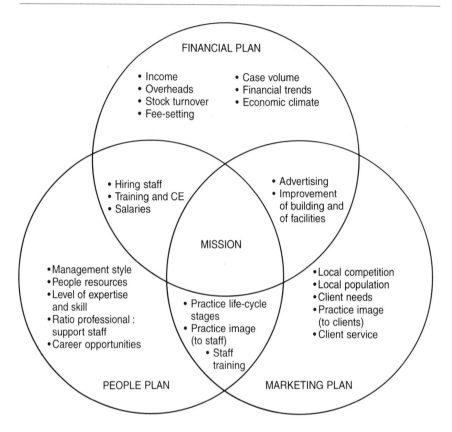

**Fig 2.1** *Planning for success: some of the factors to be considered in developing the practice's plans.*

clients seek three key benefits when they visit such a firm: expertise (the specialist), experience or efficiency. These are points along a continuous spectrum for a professional service firm; they progress from expertise to efficiency to experience to expertise. The concept of a practice life-cycle is a crude but useful model for how veterinary practice evolves. It is illustrated in Fig. 2.2 with examples of the types of veterinary practice that are found at each of the different stages.

## The efficiency practice

Clients seeking the efficiency practice are looking for routine services such as vaccinations and spays at the lowest possible cost, with the minimum of palaver. They will phone around for the cheapest price.

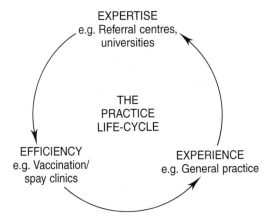

**Fig 2.2** *The practice life-cycle: examples of practices at different stages of the life-cycle.*

The efficiency practice is characterized by having a high throughput of clients, low average transaction fees (the average fee generated per client), a limited range of basic services, and a high percentage of young and relatively inexperienced staff.

Examples of efficiency practices are spay and vaccination clinics.

### The experience practice

Most clients with a sick pet would go to the experience practice where they will find a broad general knowledge of a wide variety of disease problems. These clients are neither looking for specialist skills nor, especially, to save money.

The range of services offered is much wider, the average transaction fee is higher and the throughput of clients is lower than the efficiency practice. Staff would range in skills and experience.

General practice typifies the experience practice.

### The expert practice

Clients owning an exotic pet, or one with a rare or complicated disease condition would eventually seek specialist knowledge. They expect to pay considerably more for highly individualized, expert knowledge.

These practices are characterized by having a low throughput of high-paying clients, and using only highly qualified staff. The specialist or referral practice exemplifies the expert practice.

Figure 2.3 summarizes the key differences between each type, which are expressed in more detail in Table 2.2.

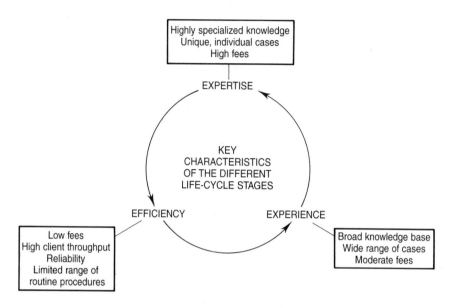

**Fig. 2.3** *Key characteristics of the stages of the practice life-cycle.*

**Table 2.2** *Important differences between the three life stages*

| Feature | Efficiency | Experience | Expertise |
|---|---|---|---|
| **What clients seek** | ■ Low cost<br>■ Speed<br>■ Reliability | ■ Broad knowledge<br>■ Good service | ■ Specialist knowledge<br>■ Highly personalized service |
| **Key characteristics** | ■ Low cost<br>■ High client throughput<br>■ Narrow range routine procedures<br>■ Low ratio vet: VN | ■ Fair fees: cost related to time<br>■ Broad range of services<br>■ Broad range of experience | ■ High fees<br>■ Each case highly individual<br>■ Narrow range very skilled procedures<br>■ Highly skilled personnel |
| **Type of work** | ■ Low risk<br>■ Routine | ■ Broad range from routine to partially specialized | ■ Highly specialized<br>■ System/discipline specific |
| **Examples of practice type** | ■ Neutering and vaccination clinics | ■ General practice | ■ Referral practice<br>■ Universities<br>■ Species - specific clinics |

**Table 2.2** *Continued*

| Feature | Efficiency | Experience | Expertise |
|---|---|---|---|
| **Ratio of professional to support staff** | ■ Low. High use of trained support staff | ■ Approx.1:2. Mixture of experienced and inexperienced staff | ■ Approx.1:2 but highly trained, specialized |
| **Ratio 'senior' to 'junior' professionals** | ■ Low: practice needs relatively simple skills and little experience | ■ Mixture: practice wants a broad knowledge base | ■ High: practice needs highly qualified 'seniors' |
| **Personnel training** | ■ Minimal for basic needs of practice | ■ Well structured and organized to disseminate information throughout practice | ■ Minimal (staff already high calibre), but very specialized |
| **Fee-setting and profitability** | ■ Fees low<br>■ Often fixed fee procedures<br>■ Dependent on high client throughput | ■ Fees fair<br>■ Profit from fee relative to time | ■ Fees high, individual<br>■ Profit per case |
| **Client throughput** | ■ High<br>■ Short appointments or 'open surgery' | ■ Moderate<br>■ 10-minute appointments<br>■ Little 'open surgery' | ■ Low<br>■ Appointment only |
| **Aims of management** | ■ Growth of business through efficiency of the individual | ■ Interdependency of practice departments to share knowledge<br>■ Professional and career development encouraged | ■ Promote quality and standards |
| **Styles of management** | ■ Tight, controlled<br>■ Emphasis on efficiency | ■ General small business management<br>■ Focus on coordination within practice | ■ Peer group consensus<br>■ Leader who symbolizes high standards |
| **Goals and growth** | ■ Rapid expansion by specific targeting | ■ Steady client base founded on sound trust relationship<br>■ Long-term commitment to improving animal health<br>■ Providing quality client service | ■ Growth not a major goal<br>■ New knowledge<br>■ Frontier science |
| **Marketing style** | ■ Heavy advertising of selected services<br>■ Target mailing | ■ Mixture: newsletters, reminders, client meetings. Based on developing trust relation | ■ Aimed at colleagues to promote perception as experts, e.g. publications, books, lectures |
| **Type of location** | ■ Multiple centres<br>■ Franchises<br>■ Individual profit centres | ■ May have branches with different characteristics | ■ One centre |
| **Professional salary** | ■ Salary scale dependent on efficiency | ■ Fixed | ■ Profit-sharing bonus system |

## How they relate to each other

When a new practice opens it is often at the efficiency stage, offering a limited range of basic services at competitively low fees. As it becomes more established it increases its range of services (e.g. it can afford to buy an X-ray machine, laboratory equipment, computer, etc.), employs staff with a wider range of experience and skills, becomes more confident about charging for services, and develops into the experience practice. After a time, individuals within the practice identify a need for specialization – they undertake extra training and the specialist or referral practice starts to emerge.

The time taken for the practice to evolve from efficiency to experience to expert depends on many factors, but is measured in years rather than months. Influencing factors include location of the practice, needs of the local market, personal and professional staff needs, and so on.

The reason that this evolution is called a life-cycle is that many of yesterday's innovative and pioneering techniques (specialist skills) eventually become tomorrow's relatively routine procedures (e.g. bitch spays, cruciate ligament repairs, aural canal ablations, cancer therapies, etc.). The link between these two, though, has the longest time span.

## Why is the practice life-cycle concept important?

Few practices have a clear picture of their true positioning along the spectrum, which is a major reason for failure of many strategic planning and practice marketing efforts within veterinary practices. Most practices try and provide all three types of service – efficiency, experience and specialist – to satisfy all their possible clients. This is partly a traditional attitude and partly muddled marketing. But each category has different aims, different managerial styles and requires different practice structuring (see Table 2.2). A practice attempting to serve too diverse a set of client needs can end up serving none of them very well, which results in dissatisfied clients and poorer standards of treatment for their animals and frustration within the practice.

The practice has the choice to go with the life-cycle, adapting and changing practice strategies as it goes, or to prevent the progression by specific actions to achieve stability.

Another option is to juggle the conflicting managerial, economic and behavioural requirements of different practice areas to combine all the different life-cycle stages. This is difficult and can only be achieved through creating artificial divisions in the practice that enable each section or branch to have its own managerial and marketing style appropriate to the market place it serves. Divisions in turn can create practical difficulties; for example, can the same vets that are the specialists maintain that expertise *and* take their turn in the duty roster for the broad experience branch of the practice? Or how can the practice weigh the demand for low-cost vaccinations against providing high quality facilities and equipment for the specialist side of the practice?

In reality, this model of life-cycle stages is over-simplistic and has to be balanced by practical considerations. The average practice in Britain is four veterinary surgeons and 10 support staff, and it would be very difficult to divide the practice into its expert, efficient and experienced sections. On the other hand, the concept of the practice life-cycle can help clarify at what stage of evolution or development the practice is now and where you want it to go. This is important when considering the next stage of business management, which is to establish a mission for the practice.

## ▉ The mission statement, goals and objectives

*Without a clear vision of where you are going and without specific behaviours to measure, it is almost impossible to achieve any goal. Goal-setting, strategies, objectives and action plans are an on-going, everchanging part of this process, and one that will be a way of life for successful enterprises from now on.*
Cannie and Caplin, Learning Dynamics, Inc.,1991

The basis of good business management is in establishing a mission, and then working to achieve that mission through strategic planning. The principle underlying strategic planning is to develop a set of actions that will make the practice's services *more valuable to clients* than the services of competing practices.

Developing a practice business strategy is a creative activity, not a purely analytical one. It is about finding new ways of doing things that provide an advantage over the competition. The practice focuses not so much on doing new things, but on doing old things differently – and better – than the competition.

Examples of this could be:

- ■ *Hiring.* Can we develop a new approach to hiring professional and support staff so that we attract a higher calibre of staff than the competition?

- *Client communication.* Can we train our staff better so that their communication skills with clients are friendlier and more helpful than the competition?
- *Client service.* Can we listen more closely to what our clients want so that we can really satisfy them with our outstanding service?

Plans are linked by the mission of the practice and are expressed in terms of objectives and goals.

- *Mission.* The basic purpose of the practice, that is, what it is trying to accomplish.
- *Objective.* A major aim of the practice which the practice will try and emphasize or develop.
- *Goal.* An objective made into a definite action plan.

Planning takes time: there is no 'quick fix' solution to running an effective business.

### Establishing a mission

A mission statement combines the requirements of three key elements of the practice: the needs of the clients, the needs of the practice personnel, and the need for success (see Fig 2.4). It is the result of a combined effort from all the members of the practice and is like the invisible hand that binds all the members of the practice together. It describes what the practice is about rather than the specific ojectives and goals the practice hopes to achieve. The mission statement is the most important step in unifying the practice.

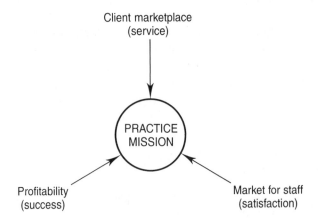

**Fig 2.4** *Components of the practice mission.*

In broad terms a typical mission would be:

> *To deliver exceptional client service; to provide professional satis-*
> *faction through fulfilling careers for our people; and to achieve*
> *financial success so that we can reward ourselves and grow.*

Writing a mission statement for the practice is not easy. It can take many months to prepare. The final mission statement should be short and succinct. It should also strive to be:

- *Feasible.* It would not be possible to combine, say, providing top quality service with rapid client throughput.
- *Motivating.* People take pride in working for organizations that are unique or different. Imagine working for a practice that said about itself, 'We are just like every other practice'!
- *Distinctive* – a common fallacy among practices is that they are automatically distinctive because of their high quality of medical and surgical care. Virtually all mission statements claim to deliver the 'highest quality' of care, but this is clearly not true and it also doesn't differentiate the practice from all the others that claim exactly the same.
- *Memorable.* The mission statement cannot be too long or complicated.

## Writing the mission statement

To define the practice mission you need to answer the following searching questions:

### What business are we in?

Veterinary practice is in the animal health care business.

### Who is our customer?

People and their animals.

### What business are we *really* in?

*i) Why do animal owners really come to our practices?*

Pritchard (1989), states that: '*Veterinary medicine is the health profession charged with the responsibility for the providing of the health needs of all kinds of animals and* **the related aspects of the health and well-being of people**.' (p. 23, my emphasis.)

In companion animal practice, clients come to veterinary practices to obtain peace of mind and relief from worry about their pets; they seek self-esteem through feeling that they are doing the right thing for their pet.

*ii) How can we express client needs in business terms?*

How can we relate their needs to the realities of managing a practice successfully? Veterinary practice is in the business of providing animal health care services to the benefit of the animals in our charge and their owners (our clients) and creating a fair profit from the transaction.

## What business *should* we be in?

This is the most difficult question to answer because it makes the practice really look at what it wants to achieve as an individual practice. It is the practice's *idealized* vision of itself. Answers should take into account factors such as the life-cycle stage of the practice, the commitment to quality client service, the role of preventive health care, the interests and experience of the practice members, and the financial objectives of the practice.

## What business *can* we be in?

Based on the practice's existing resources, skills, people, expertise, etc., this is the practice's true vision. It makes the practice relate the ideal vision to the true potential for development along the chosen strategic lines.

The practice's mission should be compatible with the personal missions of the practice principal(s) and staff (see Chapter 3 What do I want to be famous for? pp. 33–35.) to make a truly effective practice.

## ■■■ Establishing objectives

Objectives should be developed for each plan category for, say, the next 3 months, 6 months, year and long-term. They should be consistent with but separate from the mission statement. These objectives will, by necessity, vary from year to year, and will not all be compatible with each other at the same time. It is also not practical or wise to pursue all the objectives at once – it is better to grade them and work systematically through them. Too often practices attempt too much – and fail. The result is disillusionment and an unwillingness to try again – ever.

*For example, an objective for the year might be to increase practice income by 10%. This could be achieved by:*

- *Increasing the income per client; or*
- *Increasing the number of clients; or*
- *Reducing the overheads; or*
- *A combination of all three.*

*Shorter-term objectives can then be defined within this annual objective that take into consideration these three techniques, but remember it might not be feasible to, for example, increase practice income by simultaneously increasing the average transaction fee **and** increasing client throughput, or reduce overheads **and** increase the number of clients.*

## Goal formulation

Goals are objectives made into a definite plan. Of course, not all objectives will get to this stage. Goals can be expressed as SMART objectives, that is:

- Specific: what exactly is this goal?
- Measurable: Have you achieved it? How can you measure your success?
- Action-orientated: who will do it, when and how?
- Realistic: can it be achieved in the given time with the given facilities?
- Time-limited: when should it be completed or assessed?

Thus, a portion of a mission statement in a practice might read, *'We will give outstanding client service . . .'*. Some of the objectives within this practice, with an estimate of how long they should take to achieve, could be:

- To improve the telephone service (3 months).
- To widen the entrance to the practice for wheelchair and pram access (3 months).
- To develop a retail pet health care product outlet in the practice (1 year).
- To develop a range of preventive pet health care programmes (2 years).
- To enhance the role of the nurse to increase the value of inter-action with clients (6 months).

From these, a couple of SMART goals that the practice could start immediate work on could be:

- To improve the quality of the telephone service by reducing the time taken to answer the phone and the time spent on 'hold' by training reception staff in telephone skills (using an external expert), and employing part-time staff at peak periods so that the phone is answered within three rings, and the client not kept on hold longer than 1 minute. The effect of this will be measured in 3 months by direct observation of telephone staff, and through client questionnaires.
- To establish a vaccination programme that will achieve a 95% vaccination rate, measured at the end of 1 year, through use of increased client education, booster reminders, telephone contact and computerized client lists. This will primarily be the role of trained veterinary nurses.

## ■ Summary

1  Veterinary practice is in the business of serving animal owners through commitment to the health and welfare of their animals.

2  The responsive, and therefore successful, practice constantly adapts to suit the changing needs of its market – animal owners and their animals.

3  The key to business success is planning. Planning gives direction and control.

4  Planning starts by identifying which stage of the practice life-cycle the practice is in – expertise, efficiency or experience.

5  Next, the practice needs to define a mission and work out the objectives and goals needed to achieve that mission.

6  Finally, the practice needs to plan the development of the three major practice areas – finance, marketing and people.

# 3 Leadership and Management

*A leader is there to disturb the status quo*

WHAT is it that distinguishes the responsive practice from the average? Is it having a modern building? A good marketing policy? Lots of new ideas? Is it a feature of the number of veterinarians in the practice? Whilst many factors may contribute to success, the one characteristic shared by the responsive practices that I believe is the most important is the outstanding skills and behaviour of the practice leader(s).

Do practices need leaders? After all, they are peopled by intelligent, energetic individuals whom it should be possible to rely upon to be self-managing, high achievers. The simple answer is, 'Yes'. Both professional and support staff in practices lead busy lives with many conflicting demands on their time and attention. They often become so involved with the minutiae of the present that they lose sight of where they want to go with their lives. Good practice leaders provide the direction and drive to help their staff accomplish more and greater things than they would do on their own. This simultaneously builds a happier and more productive practice.

## The importance of being 'focused'

Without exception, the leaders of the responsive practices that I know are well 'focused': they have clearly identified what they want to be and what they want to do, and they have established the values or principles on which this being and doing are based. By being focused they have become *effective* (see Table 3.1: Effective versus efficient). By being effective they achieve more of what they really need to do.

**Table 3.1** *Effectiveness vs. efficiency*

**Effectiveness** is doing the right things well. It is the goal of a leader.

**Efficiency** is doing things well, but not necessarily the right ones. A leader is needed to ensure the right things are being done.

> *For example, a team may be very efficiently repairing the small hole in the bows of a sinking ship, but the water that's going to sink the ship is pouring in through the gash in the stern. The effective set of actions in this case would be to fix the hole in the stern.*

## ■■■ What characterizes an effective practice leader?

> *As a business leader there is one thing you can count on as you move through the nineties: change. Your success as a leader will be based upon your ability to adapt, respond and bend to the conditions around you.*
> Bradford and Raines, Management Consultants

Personal characteristics these leaders have in common are a willingness to work hard, decisiveness, enthusiasm, and, perhaps most important of all, an ability to adapt quickly to change. But these characterize what they *are* rather than what they *do* – and it is their ability to get things *done* which is what makes them such outstanding leaders. They are not afraid to start new things, to show others the way forward and to positively influence the people with whom they work.

## ■■■ Surely all practice principals are leaders?

Practice principals are typically dedicated clinicians, primarily interested in animal care, who seek the autocracy of independence from being an employee. They have to assume leadership as an integral part of practice ownership but most lack commitment to leadership; they don't want to take on (and don't know what is involved in) the full responsibility of leadership. As a result, most principals bury their heads, ostrich-like, in the sands of clinical work and hope that all the administrative, financial and personnel problems will resolve themselves.

## ■■■ So, what are practice principals?

In most practices, principals have to be multi-faceted. They have to be leaders, managers, practice owners and veterinarians: different roles requiring different skills. For the principals of smaller practices, there is often no reasonably viable alternative.

A *leader* gets things done through people by making meaning for them and a desire to achieve. A leader is *effective*. He or she requires good communication, negotiation, delegation and self-management skills, coupled with long-term perspective.

A *manager* creates the environment in which people can be more effective. A manager is *efficient*. A manager's time is more splintered than a leader's with a greater diversity of problems and situations to deal with in any one day, and the results are more ambiguous and difficult to measure.

An *owner* is most interested in the practice's *profit*.

A *clinical veterinarian* concentrates on the diagnosis, treatment and management of the consultations, operations and visits booked. His or her day ends with visible signs of progress which can be measured in a number of different ways, such as number of clients seen, and income generated.

These are all different behaviours, different expectations and different measures of progress and achievement: trying to combine these contrasting roles can only result in compromise for the multi-faceted principal.

## ■■■ Can principals learn to be better leaders?

Yes, but they have to decide what aspect of multi-faceted principalship they want to focus on and delegate much of the rest in the practice. Unfortunately, most principals are afraid of losing authority through delegation and prefer to 'do it all themselves'. This is not necessarily what is best for the practice.

Practice principals are, first and foremost, veterinarians. Their primary – and economic – strength is as clinical veterinarians. They have no training as leaders/managers/owners responsible for the financial success of a business. Their value to the practice may be far lower in these secondary roles.

The decision that has to be made within the practice is how is the practice principal most *valuable* to the practice? In which role(s) does he or she become more of an overhead than a valuable production unit? Which role(s) should be developed? (See also later, How should you spend your time? page 35)

What are the alternatives for a multi-faceted principal?

## Clinician with a vision

To become a 'clinician with a vision' a practice principal could hire a manager. By delegating the responsibility for the day-to-day running of the practice to a suitably qualified person the principal can continue to perform the clinical work he or she is so skilled at (and contribute most effectively to the practice income), *and* be able to have the vision that takes the practice forward and makes it special. (However, see the section on practice managers below.)

## A question of ownership

At the moment, only veterinary surgeons are allowed to own private practices. The Royal College of Veterinary Surgeons regards it as *'undesirable, both from a professional and a public point of view, that any veterinarian in the conduct of a private practice should be subject to the direction and control of a lay person or persons'* (RCVS Guide to Professional Conduct, 1993, section 17.5.1, p. 54). But there is a marked trend away from veterinarians *wanting* to own their own practices. The heavy financial and personal commitment involved is felt by many to offer inadequate return, even in the long term.

In other European countries, such as Sweden, lay ownership of veterinary practices, or at least guidance by a board of non-veterinarian directors, is acceptable. As long as careful, established guidelines for professional behaviour and standards are followed, this can enhance the business potential and efficiency of the practice by using the skills and experiences of people from other professions and businesses. Lay ownership or direction frees the practice principal for what he or she is most valuable as – being a veterinarian.

## Reality?

The most likely way in the immediately forseeable future for practice principals to enhance their multi-faceted roles and make themselves more effective is to learn to focus themselves, show their staff how to become focused and more effective, and to use better time management. This can be summarized in one word – *planning*. Practice principals need to plan their own professional life and help plan their staff's lives in the context of the practice mission.

Other leadership skills, such as improved communication, motivation and delegation skills, can also be learnt or enhanced (see Chapter 7 for their practical application).

## What do I want to be famous for?

Veterinarians are typically highly trained, intelligent and usually ambitious people. They want to feel special and feel that the practice they belong to is special. But remarkably few are focused.

It is difficult to focus, to write down your personal mission or creed: what it is that will make you special. But by being focused and by having a clear sense of direction in your life, you become more effective; you achieve more and gain greater satisfaction from life than those who merely drift.

One method to help you focus is to ask yourself, 'What do I want to be famous for?', i.e. 'What do I want to do in my life that will make me special?'.

It will actually be fairly difficult to define the answers clearly and precisely, and it may take some months before you are able to do so. The answers can sometimes be quite surprising. Once you have defined them, work out the steps you need to take to achieve them, and a time plan for each step. Be brave! Challenge yourself! – don't limit yourself with self-imposed constraints.

## What do my staff want to be famous for?

Leaders get things done through people, but the people need to know what they want to do – and what they need to do to help the business they are in. A practice leader helps his people achieve both the practice vision and their own, vision-compatible goals.

Ask each member of staff what they want to be famous for – and help them find the answer. By making them clarify their ambitions, you create a team of people that is ready to work for the practice vision and simultaneously grow their own individual skills and abilities. The effect of focusing your staff is illustrated in Figs 3.1 and 3.2.

In the unfocused practice (Fig. 3.1) people (A–F) are not working effectively because they don't know either what the practice stands for or what they want from their lives.

In the focused practice (Fig. 3.2), A–D have personal missions that are

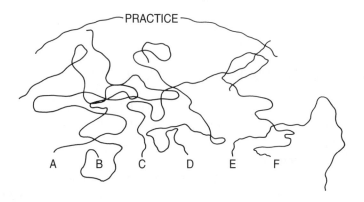

**Fig. 3.1** *The unfocused practice.*

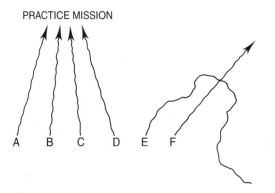

**Fig. 3.2** *The focused practice. A–D have personal missions in line with the practice mission, E remains unfocused, F's mission is not in line with the practice mission, so he or she will probably leave.*

compatible with the practice mission; they will grow and develop as the practice develops. Character E cannot focus and will continue to be undetermined and ineffective. Character F finds that the practice mission is not compatible with his or her own aims (perhaps to work in a different type of practice, go into research or industry, or learn particular skills that he or she cannot get from the practice) so they would be best to leave and find a more suitable practice for their needs. If they remain they will be dissatisfied and resentful which could affect the work performance of others in the practice.

## ▰▰ Improving your effectivity through time management

### *Why is time management so important?*

Poor time management is a sign of disorganization and is the limiting factor to effectivity (Drucker, 1966). You have only 24 hours in a day. There are a certain number of jobs and procedures you are required to complete in that time, plus dealing with the general problems that arise daily in practice. Much time-wasting comes from an inability to set priorities and stick to them. By planning and organizing your time you *can* achieve all you want and more. Not only will you have more time to pursue other interests and hobbies, but you can also retain your enthusiasm for and enjoyment of practice life.

### *So how should you spend your time?*

There are numerous ways in which to manage time better detailed in a variety of self-help manuals. Some common time-wasters and a simple guide to making better use of your time are outlined in Tables 3.2 and 3.3.

However, the multi-faceted principal requires a time management plan which highlights the relative importance of each of his various roles, controls the time spent on each, and makes that time as effective as possible.

**Table 3.2** *Common time-wasters*

- Long/unscheduled telephone calls
- Interruptions
- Unnecessary meetings
- Handling the daily mail
- Poor office desk management
- Poor medical records/record filing system
- Inability to say 'no'
- Poorly managed appointment system with unscheduled appointments
- Inability to delegate
- Poor use of trained support staff

**Table 3.3** *Improve your time management*

1    Start by recording how your time is spent. Compare it with your idea of how you spend your time.

2    Cut back on unproductive use of time by managing your time, i.e. making yourself accountable for all the time you have.

   ■ Take 10 seconds to ask yourself:
       Why am I doing this?
       Who else could do it?
       Does it need to be done at all?
       What priority does it deserve?
   ■ Identify and eliminate all things that need not be done at all, i.e. that are a pure waste of time leading to no results.
   ■ Delegate jobs that could be done as well or better by other members of the practice.
   ■ Avoid wasting other people's time, and thence your own, e.g. on long meetings.
   ■ Don't plan too tightly – allow some reactive time for events which are beyond your control (e.g. travel time between farm visits, 'breathing space' between meetings, etc.). *This can be as much as 10% of your day.*

3    Consolidate your time into the largest possible units – it is impossible to work effectively in little dribs and drabs.

   ■ Know your limits, e.g. your effective time span, your most productive working time.
   ■ Keep control of your time plan, don't be sidetracked from it by minor issues.
   ■ Improve your effectiveness by making lists of what you want to achieve that day, with priority ranking. Don't be sidetracked from these.

4    Make sure other members of your practice know about and understand your time plan so that they can co-operate with you. For example, in Swedish veterinary practices, most veterinarians have a fixed daily telephone time during which they deal with all telephone queries from clients. For this system to work, staff must know when that time is, and channel calls to the veterinarian during that time. Similarly, if you decide to do your clinical work 3 days a week, and the other days are for administration, etc., make sure your staff know about it.

*A leader's success is measured through his people's achievements.* Maister (1993) identifies the most important role of a practice leader as coaching and encouraging staff to fulfil their potential. I have adapted his time plan (for the principals of legal firms) to the requirements of veterinary principals as follows:

- *Administration*: not more than 10% time. If it takes more time than this to keep abreast of paperwork, hire a trained administrator.
- *Clinical work*: not more than 20%. For a truly effective practice *leader*, performing clinical work is *not* the most productive use of time but it may be necessary to maintain professional respect. (However, see earlier – the problem of the multi-faceted principal – clinician. In addition, in a small practice the proportion of time spent on clinical work must, by necessity, be much higher.)
- *Marketing and selling*: not more than 10%. It is not the job of the practice leader to promote the practice through client meetings, organizing the practice marketing, and so on, although it is important that the leader fully supports practice marketing. This role can be delegated to suitably trained staff.
- *General client relations*: not more than 20%. A certain amount of time solving client problems and, more importantly, canvassing clients for their ideas, comments and criticisms is invaluable but should not take more than a fifth of the total time.
- *Coaching veterinary surgeons and staff:* up to 60%. The most productive use of a *leader's* time lies in individual coaching to get the best from staff members. By helping staff solve their problems, keep their priorities straight, and set themselves stretching goals, coach–leaders enable the individuals in the practice to achieve more than they would on their own – which has the added advantage of improving the practice's productivity too. Coaching is not easy: changing peoples ways of working and doing things is hard because people prefer to stick to what they know and feel comfortable with, and because different individuals are motivated by different things.

    A good coach structures small, simple changes, with which it is easy to attain success, and which give people confidence to try new things. They also work hard to develop joint tasks so that staff gain the experience of teamwork and joint responsibility. The practice becomes much more effective if the staff function as a team rather than a group (see Chapters 5 and 6).

This time plan would have to modified for the principal of a small practice but it still provides, I believe, a useful indicator of how leaders should best focus their time.

## ■ A final word about leadership

There is no easy answer to the problem of how to make practice principals better, more effective business leaders, but much of the solution lies with the principals themselves. To be truly effective as *leaders* they need to learn new skills of people and self management. For many principals, this is not what they want to do.

Think carefully about your various roles as practice principal. Where are you *really* most valuable to the practice? What do you *truly* enjoy doing most? Be honest with yourself. Look at the options available for yourself and the practice. Hiring a full-time practice manager? Remaining an assistant/salaried partner? Taking time to train and develop new professional leadership skills? Studying for an MBA? Work out what is best for you and your practice.

## ■ Where do practice managers fit in?

Although the terms leader and manager are regarded by many authors as being synonymous (and in veterinary practice are often the same person), 'pure' leaders and managers have different actions and aims. They require the same basic skills in:

- planning;
- budgeting;
- organizing;
- controlling.

In addition, a 'pure' leader must have:

- an ability to invent and apply suitable motivators;
- an ability to inspire;
- a strong vision of the future that incorporates the long-term interests of everyone involved;
- clear, deep-seated values upon which every decision is founded.

The leader/manager relationship has been likened to a group hacking their way through the jungle: the manager, who typically works by rational, applied means, ensures they are hacking efficiently, but it is the visionary leader who climbs the tallest tree and makes sure they are in the right jungle.

## ■■■ What is the role of the manager in veterinary practice?

A manager's role is to get things done, achieve goals, and get results. For this, maturity, experience and authority are essential. A truly effective manager should have the authority to, for example, hire and fire both professional and support staff, to evaluate and coach staff and reward performance, to train support staff, to control drug and equipment purchase, to maintain the practice, work with book-keeping, accounting and legal issues, have financial accountability for the practice and do the banking, and have responsibility for miscellaneous duties such as maintaining strict standards for cleanliness, and updating the practice library.

Sheridan and McCafferty (1993) define three, graded levels of management that apply in veterinary practice:

- *The office manager* – who is responsible for implementing and co-ordinating the administrative directions determined by the practice owner or hospital director.
- *The practice manager* – who has greater responsibilities than the office manager which may include the overall co-ordination of financial activities, preparation of budgets, hiring and firing of support staff, and generally having more authority for the day-to-day running of the practice. They are still answerable to the practice owner(s).
- *The practice or hospital administrator* – a qualified, experienced person with complete authority over the running of the practice. Apart from clinical matters, he or she is responsible for every aspect of practice activity.

Most practices have not progressed beyond having an office manager.

## ■■■ Some reasons why practice managers are not successful – yet!

*Good practice managers are rare, but so is a practice that will tolerate a good practice manager.*
Don Dooley, Veterinary Management Consultant, 1992

Practice managers can make a very significant difference to the productivity of a practice but for many principals the abdication of authority that ownership of the practice entails to a better-qualified third party is an almost impossible hurdle to overcome and, as a result, so-called practice managers are very limited in what they can achieve. Until veterinarians have the self-confidence to truly hand over these responsibilites to a practice manager, the best that can be achieved in most practices is learning to delegate the many duties a good practice manager could undertake to suitably trained staff members.

## Guide to Professional Conduct

The RCVS Guide to Professional Conduct, 1993 states:

> **17.5.1** *'It is undesirable both from a professional and a public point of view, that any veterinarian in the conduct of a private practice should be subject to the direction and control of a lay person or persons. It follows that where a practice manager is employed, he must exercise no control over clinical matters.'* (p.54)

This is often interpreted literally by veterinarians to mean that the manager can have almost no authority: some are hardly more than office-juniors.

## Veterinarian versus practice manager!

Veterinarians resent taking advice from non-veterinarians. However, for a (non-veterinarian) manager to be effective he must have the authority to control the productivity of the veterinarians on the staff, including the productivity of the practice principal(s). If the authority is not given – and most practice owners baulk at the idea of being advised what to do – then the manager's effectivity is immediately drastically reduced.

In many practices the practice manager is a non-veterinarian who has either been promoted from a nursing or reception position, or is retired from a civilian position (bank manager, accountant, etc.). Of the former group, many do not have the maturity and confidence based on experience and understanding of the requirements of their role to exert the necessary authority; the latter are seldom given the necessary authority.

Some practices hire a retired veterinarian or retain a semi-retired partner as the practice manager. Although these practitioners may bring a wealth of clinical experience with them, they can have a negative effect on practice development in a number of ways:

- They retain old-fashioned ideas and policies and are not receptive to new ideas.
- Their skills are as clinicians not managers.
- They are less financially productive as managers than when using their clinical skills (but often still expect a high salary commensurate with their clinical experience).
- They do not necessarily have the people management skills essential for the job.

Another source of practice managers is the principal's non-veterinarian spouse. This may seem the ideal solution in a small practice; for example, the boss's spouse can take the load of responsibility for all the non-clinical procedures in the practice. In reality, the close relationship of the manager to the practice owner often creates many problems:

- Staff are afraid/feel unable to come to the manager to discuss problems concerning the boss, or vice versa.
- The manager is felt to have undue influence over the boss which may spill over into management of clinical aspects of the practice.
- The manager may abuse the position of authority and make employees' lives very difficult.

Practices like this are often characterized by a high turnover of unhappy professional and support staff.

## Is there a future for practice managers?

*Because most practices are still owned by a veterinarian or veterinarians who work in the practice, true practice management will probably be a rare position for the forseeable future.*
Don Dooley, Veterinary Management Consultant

Yes. Since Dooley's rather negative statement was made, the attitude towards the veterinary practice manager has changed considerably. Responsive practices already recognize the value of true practice managers, and employ them to a significant extent.

More and better education courses are becoming available for veterinary practice managers all the time. Bristol University, for example, has started a modular course for veterinary surgeons and those directly concerned with different management aspects of veterinary practice, and Certificates are available in subjects such as accounting, and general management. The

British Veterinary Practice Managers Association is currently formulating a certification programme for its members, which will be at post-graduate level, and is very active in promoting 'hands on' practice management to practitioners and their staff. I believe it will not be long before managers can assume a much greater role in veterinary practice.

## ■ Summary

1 Responsive practices have strong leaders.

2 The multi-faceted leader (who attempts to combine being a leader with being a manager, owner and veterinary clinician) can become much more effective by:

  ■ learning to focus;
  ■ using time management;
  ■ coaching staff.

3 Practice managers contribute enormously to the running of the practice – if they are allowed to.

# 4 Improving Communication in Veterinary Practice

*Human beings carry an ability to receive, interpret and emotionally distort every message they receive.*

Hayes and Watts, Business Management Consultants

COMMUNICATION is something that everyone does every day on many different levels and yet communication problems are the greatest cause of stress, job dissatisfaction, and disappointed clients in veterinary practice. Good communication is critically important because it is the foundation of a healthy business.

Responsive practices have learnt the value of good communication at the two primary levels: internally (between staff and with colleagues) and externally (with clients). Although the basic *principles* of communication are the same with either group, the aims and outcomes are different (see Table 4.1).

These issues are explored in more depth in this chapter where I present some important general information about communication techniques and how to enhance them. In the next chapter, some of the issues behind poor interpersonnel and staff–client relations are examined, and ways are suggested to overcome these and thus create a happier practice environment

**Table 4.1** *Communicating with colleagues and clients*

| Methods | Purpose | Results |
| --- | --- | --- |
| Voice and words | Create trust | ***Staff/colleagues*** |
| Active listening | Convey interest, care | Happy, productive, |
| Body language | and concern | creative work |
| Written material and | Convey professionalism | environment |
| visual aids | | ***Clients*** |
| Touch | | Repeat business, income |
| (Smell) | | Better animal health |

and more satisfied clients. Communication is a vast subject and for the sake of clarity and brevity I have selected those aspects of communication which I believe are most important.

# What is communication?

Communication is the sharing or exchange of information, ideas, or feelings. It is a complex learned skill which uses all the senses (sight, hearing, touch, smell and taste). It is also central to good business.

# Communication techniques

### Voice and words

In a face-to-face meeting less than 40% of the exchange depends on the words being spoken; most information for the receiver comes from non-verbal signals such as tone of voice, facial expression, eye contact, and body language. A cold, brusque voice is alienating, and a shrill, loud voice can be both irritating and wearing. The ideal voice is warm, friendly and fairly low-pitched.

Voice is especially important on the telephone where the caller cannot see the person and makes a judgement from voice alone. Less than 15% of the impression made on the telephone comes from the words spoken. How the words are said (tone of voice, pitch, speed) can be positively influenced by smiling as you talk, and using gestures. As you are using only your auditory sense, good listening skills become critical.

### Active listening

Equally important for the effective exchange of information in a conversation is active listening. It is estimated that we use less than 25% of our listening powers in a typical exchange and ignore, forget, distort or misunderstand a staggering 75%. This creates frustration (e.g. from not listening to the nurse who suggests a valuable time-saving technique), loses business (not hearing the client who mentions that Bonzo has intermittent diarrhoea, a condition which might respond to dietary or medical management), and may even be dangerous (not hearing the client who says that Fluffy is drinking more, which may mean diagnostic blood tests for renal disease are advisable before giving the anaesthetic for the dental you'd planned).

Active listening is just that: listening actively, paying full attention to the speaker, and digesting and interpreting the true meaning of what is being said. It conveys respect ('I think highly enough of your opinion and views to want to listen to them'), and is the bridge to understanding. It is also hard work (see Table 4.2).

It is difficult to talk to somebody who is apparently not responding and may create feelings of confusion, anger and discomfort on the part of the speaker that stop further communication. By using encouraging body language (such as nodding your head), eye contact, facial and auditory signals ('Yes, I see'; 'Mmmm, that's interesting') coupled with repeating or paraphrasing what the person has said ('If I understand you correctly, you think that Tibbles . . .'; 'Jim, from what you've just said, the problem with the current X-ray system is . . .') you indicate that you understand and are interested in what the speaker is saying. On the telephone where people can't see you nodding and agreeing with them, make agreeing noises ('Yes', 'Ah-ha', 'I see . . .' and so on).

### Body language

Body language is an integral part of face-to-face communication. It is generally an involuntary and therefore truthful indicator of what the speaker is actually thinking, whatever words he or she may be choosing to use. Body language involves the whole body, from the spatial position one person adopts in relation to another, through arm and hand gestures, to barely perceptible movements of the facial muscles.

Closed body language (crossed arms, looking away from the person to whom you are speaking, turning your back) shows disinterest, and lack of receptivity. Many people sense this and are put off by it. Staff may feel, 'The boss wasn't really interested in my problem', and clients may

**Table 4.2** *Common barriers to listening and understanding*

- Hearing unfamiliar words
- Speaking too fast
- Doing other things simultaneously/distractions
- Excess background noise
- 'Switching off'
- Being critical
- Being compliant for the sake of comfort
- Using an inappropriate or incorrect form of address
- Tiredness

comment to their friends, 'That vet wasn't really interested – he didn't listen to me'. Table 4.3 gives ways of improving body language.

Open body language, and mirroring or copying body language signals help break down barriers to communication. Copying body language conveys a very important non-verbal message. It tells others you like them or agree with them, and vice versa (Pease, 1984). Professional salespeople are taught to use strong body language – observe how their body language influences you and your interpretation of what they are saying.

**Table 4.3** *Simple ways to improve your body language*

- Smile when you meet the client
- Shake hands when the client enters the consulting room
- Fondle their pet and show kindness to it
- Have a friendly, welcoming expression
- Look interested in what the client is saying
- Maintain the 'open position' (avoid crossing your arms in front of you, or sitting with your arms and legs crossed
- Avoid turning your back on your client
- Maintain at least 60% eye contact during a conversation
- Don't fiddle with things or glance at your watch – it implies lack of interest
- Have clean hands and nails and keep your hands out of your pockets
- Take pride in your professional appearance
- Avoid habits such as nail-biting, hair-twisting, etc. – they are distracting

## Use of written material and visual aids

Visual aids are a very important part of communication between human beings because man is primarily a visual creature. Studies of patients visiting human medical doctors have shown that patients retain less than 10% of everything discussed in the consulting room immediately afterwards. Assuming our clients have the same retentive powers there is clearly more we can do to get information across. Information sheets, newsletters, and written instructions will help to reinforce and enhance the verbal message (see Appendix 2 for further information on using promotional material). In addition, there is often an innate acceptance of the written word whereas the reliability of the spoken word may be questioned.

Writing something down helps clarify the information to be conveyed, and reduces the opportunities for misinterpretation. Clearly written job descriptions, signed agendas from meetings and written protocols are therefore essential to good communication within the practice.

> *Beware the pointed memo though! A colleague once worked in a practice where the practice manager sent everyone frequent, hand-scribbled memos, always marked Urgent!. The result was irritation and lack of co-operation amongst the staff.*

Slides, overheads, whiteboards, models, diagrams and sections of skeletons aid explanations and presentations to colleagues and clients alike.

### Touch

Although there are many complex social taboos surrounding touch and physical contact, touch is still a very important part of communication. A welcoming handshake, or a comforting arm around the shoulders of a grieving client can say far more than words alone.

### Smell

The importance of smell is also underestimated particularly as part of the 'first impressions' a client gains of the practice (see Chapter 5, p. 62). What impression does a client gain of a practice where the receptionist wears an overpowering scent, or the veterinarian smells unwashed, or the practice reeks of tom cat urine? After all, what are your reactions to the client who has powerful halitosis, or smells of drink, or owns a poodle soaked in expensive scent?

People's sensitivity to smells does vary, but never underestimate the effect a smell can have on a person.

## Barriers to communication

The major barrier to communication is our very natural tendency to judge, evaluate, approve or disapprove of what the other person is saying. Because the human mind processes words at four times the rate we speak or hear them we often think we understand the other person before we have heard them out.

Other barriers to communication which can profoundly reduce its effectiveness are:

- *Hearing what you want to hear* – what we hear and understand is largely based on personal experience and background. We have many preconceived notions and ideas so that we often hear what our mind *thinks* a person has said, not what they actually *have* said.

- *Ignoring conflicting information* – we often choose to ignore or forget information that does not concur with our own beliefs.

- *Perceptions about the communicator* – we are often more accepting of someone we like, even if what they say is wrong, than someone we innately dislike.

- *Influence of the group* – the group with which we identify influences our attitudes and feelings, thus we are far more likely to listen and accept the words of a fellow veterinarian than those of someone outside the field.

- *The meaning of words* – words mean different things to different people. A simple example is 'chronic': in medical terms it means a long-term condition (e.g. 'He has chronic hepatitis'), whereas in layman's terms it means something not very pleasant, rather dreary (e.g. 'It was a chronic party', 'He's really chronic').

- *Non-verbal communication* – body language can convey a very different message from the verbal one, or it can support it. Sometimes, body language is all that is needed to convey a meaning; for example, a client wordlessly bursting into tears when told their pet is very ill, or biting their nails nervously while waiting for an appointment.

- *Emotions* – our emotions often cloud our interpretation of messages. For example, if we are worried and anxious we are less able to concentrate and accept ideas; if we are angry we may be totally intolerant of otherwise perfectly good suggestions. Appreciating how emotions can be a barrier to understanding is especially important when talking to the owner of a very ill or dying pet. They may be so upset they are unable to make rational and sensible decisions, and you may have to repeat things several times before they 'sink in'.

- *Practice size* – the bigger the practice and the more people in it, the greater the chance of misunderstandings and miscommunications arising. As practices get larger, managers need to take greater and greater care that communication remains clear.

# ■ Some important general points about improving communication

### *Creating trust*

> *... Trust isn't something you can mandate, a lever you can simply pull to improve an organization. Trust is an* **outcome**, *something that develops gradually in organizations that are well designed and well led. To say ... 'Now we must all trust one another' is to say nothing at all.*
> J. Richard Hackman, Harvard Professor of Psychology

A healthy trust relationship between colleagues and with clients is the basis for a sound business. Establishing trust takes time and determination. Trust comes from many little actions, rather than one or two big ones. It is very precious; once lost it takes a very long time to re-establish.

Trust can be created by always showing courtesy, kindness and honesty, keeping commitments, conveying an 'I care' attitude, and maintaining professional and personal integrity at all times by matching your actions to your words and treating everyone by the same set of values.

Trust is the highest form of human motivation; it brings out the best in people. By allowing colleagues plenty of scope for professional development, and supporting and encouraging that development without jealousy, and by working to develop staff competency to get the best from staff rather than accepting mediocrity, practice members can rise to the level of trust put in them.

Creating trust with clients comes from a willingness to help clients. It starts by having an agreed policy in the practice that the client is the most valued member of the practice. Where the client is regarded as a mere intrusion on the day, trust can never develop satisfactorily. Trust comes from listening to clients and hearing what they are *really* saying, and taking every opportunity to help them take better care of their pets through the use of recommended professional services and products

### *Conveying professionalism*

A professional attitude means wanting to serve people to the best of your ability within your professional capacity. Like many professionals, veterinarians often have a somewhat arrogant attitude: 'We are the best. Our clients should automatically recognize that'. Professional arrogance is no longer an acceptable way of running business; serving people, and seeking to help them is the way forward.

Professionalism is the manner in which a professional conducts him or herself. For most people, professionalism is, at least initially, judged by appearance, so it is foolish to think that experience and ability is automatically communicated whatever you look like. Attention to professional dress helps convey the message that colleagues and clients alike are dealing with a qualified, competent veterinary professional.

> *For example, the head of a top human surgical spinal referral clinic, who prefers to dress casually in jeans and a sweatshirt, found that this image was totally unacceptable when he was trying to establish a new market for the clinic across Europe. Prospective clients wanted their surgeon to **look** like a top professional which meant a collar and tie, good quality trousers and polished shoes, under a spotless white coat.*

Adopt a professional dress code throughout the practice: for example the British Veterinary Nursing Association has a uniform code for their trainee and full members. Other support staff can also wear co-ordinating uniforms. This serves several functions. Uniforms:

- look smart and professional;
- give a consistent feel to the practice (this *is* ABC Vet Clinic);
- help clients know who is who in a clinic;
- give the staff members a feeling of belonging;
- define 'work time' as different from 'personal time';
- help protect own clothes;
- avoid the problem of staff wearing unsuitable clothes to work.

Use lapel labels with the staff member's name, qualification and position (e.g. veterinary surgeon, veterinary nurse, receptionist, practice manager, etc.) clearly printed on. It is arrogance to assume clients know who you are and what your role is in the practice.

Convey professionalism through communicating quality at every step of the way. This is the challenge of the modern practice. Communicating quality, or marketing, starts from the moment the client tries to contact the practice and continues as they drive into the car park, enter the building, sit in the reception area, meet the veterinarian, collect their pet after an operation, and so on (see Chapter 11 for detailed information on practice marketing and the effective communication of services). Communicating quality is a constant, ongoing process.

# ▆▆▆ Improving telephone skills*

### ▆▆▆ *Why are telephone skills so important?*

The telephone is often the first contact with the practice. The person answering the phone represents the practice. They must 'sell' the practice by voice alone, and are responsible for creating some of the very first 'moments of truth' in the practice. This telephone response can literally win or lose clients, and thus business.

The telephone is both a best friend and a worst enemy. It is the essential contact with the outside world, but it can also be a very real time trap. Improving the telephone service is part of good client service to which everyone in the practice should be committed.

### ▆▆▆ *What are telephone skills?*

Telephone skills are:

- The ability to behave courteously, politely and efficiently during any telephone interaction.
- The ability to create business both directly (e.g. an appointment) or indirectly (e.g. good will) thus using the telephone as an effective marketing tool.
- Ensuring time spent on the telephone is productive and not wasted. Wasted time represents wasted money for the practice (ineffectual use of staff time, telephone bills) and can be a source of irritation and frustration to your clients.

### ▆▆▆ *Standard answering technique*

A good answering technique that everyone in the practice is trained to use helps communicate an image to the client of a quality team of efficient, service-oriented animal care professionals, and gives an excellent start to a relationship. A well-proven standard method is:

- Answer promptly within three rings – apologise to the caller if it takes longer than this to answer.
- Adopt a pleasant helpful, positive and efficient attitude.
- Greet the caller, identify the practice and yourself by name, and ask how you may help the caller.
- Screen the call and deal with the query: for example book an appointment, give the necessary advice, refer to the person requested, etc.

---

* This section first appeared in *The Veterinary Business Journal* (1994) **4**, 22–25.

- Never treat any call as routine – to the caller this particular call may be very important.
- If appropriate, write the owner's name (address), telephone number, pet's name, sex, nature of problem and other relevant details as a memo to deal with later. Read the details back to the caller to make sure you have them correctly.
- If it is necessary to put the caller on hold, ask them if it is convenient first, then check back with them every 20–30 seconds to ensure they know they are not forgotten. Apologize for keeping them waiting.
- At the end of the call, check that you have answered all their questions, and thank the caller for phoning.

### *Improving the service*

*I phoned a consumer advisory agency and asked for a Miss Smith. The receptionist told me she was off sick. Could anyone else help me with my problem? I asked, and explained briefly what it was. No, she answered. When should I try contacting Miss Smith again? When she's better, I was told. You can imagine my level of satisfaction with the firm – but I have also phoned veterinary practices and had similar responses from receptionists!*

Some pointers to improving the telephone service you currently offer include:

- Ensure *everyone* in the practice follows the same basic telephone technique.
- Have *memo pads and pens fixed* near the telephone so that they are readily accessible.
- Have a *reference folder* near the telephone at all times which gives the answers to common questions and outlines practice protocol on common proceedings (see Appendix 1).
- While the client is on hold, *use a message* on the answer machine which gives details of the services offered by the practice.
- Have a *timer* next to the phone and restrict calls to 3–5 minutes.
- *Train* all staff in answering technique. Monitor the effect of their training by tapping calls (with their knowledge) and discussing them with them.
- Use *simple language* and do not use slang.

- *Think about your choice of words*: 'Fluffy has settled into the ward' sounds much better than 'Fluffy's sitting in her cage'.
- Use the *client's name* during the call.
- Do not make *personal calls* where clients can see or hear you. Use a private line for personal calls.
- Ensure *adequate staffing* at peak times.
- If you have to *phone a client back,* do it within the agreed time.
- Where relevant, send *information* sheets to the client rather than wasting time explaining lengthy procedures over the phone. Follow this up with a phone call a few days later to see if you can help them further.
- *Price quotations* given over the phone should always be recorded (on the client's record card with a signature and date) unless they are for fixed price items or procedures.
- To improve efficiency, *plan* what you are going to say, and get references you may need to use to hand, before you make an outgoing call.
- Consider developing a *special line* for veterinary telephone advice that clients pay for directly.
- Develop *client questionnaires* to identify the best and worst aspects of your current telephone service, and to give a base to work from in improving your standards. *Regularly reassess* your telephone service as part of your overall service to clients.

### Using the telephone as a marketing tool

Some callers are just shopping around for the best price. They can be converted to loyal clients by a well-trained receptionist. A conversation can be extended to take an interest in the client and gain a commitment from them. The receptionist must portray value and a caring image by voice alone. The following guidelines can turn a phone shopper into a client:

- Greet the caller.
- Before answering the caller's question about price of a service, ask them about their pet – name, age, breed, vaccinal history. Be friendly and interested.
- Tell the caller what this practice offers and why it is unique. Explain why your services are the best for her and her pet. Keep cost at a low profile – sell the client the benefits of your services. It may be appropriate to send information through the post, but phone and see if it answered her queries a few days later.

- Make the appointment.
- Reaffirm your interest in the client and their pet by saying you look forward to seeing them on the specified day.
- Thank them for calling.

## Acknowledgement

The section on improving telephone skills first appeared as 'Improving your telephone service' in *Veterinary Business Journal* 4, December 1994, pp. 22–25.

## Summary

1   Communication is an integral and complex part of human inter- action and involves all the senses.

2   Far more than words are used to convey meaning.

3   It is possible to improve communication by concentrating on skills such as active listening, and using written and visual support material.

4   The telephone is an important business tool which maintains and builds business.

# 5 Improving People Relations

*People recognize the need to communicate but find it difficult. Like Schopenhauer's hedgehogs, they want to get together, it's only their prickles that keep them apart.*

Michael Armstrong, Management Consultant

A GOOD communication system within the practice creates a team of well-organized, happy staff who are willing to help their clients. The more trust that is developed between staff and clients through good communication, the more co-operation and success the practice will experience.

A client visiting a practice expects professional levels of medical and surgical care, but can only measure that professionalism in terms of the service they receive. Excellent communication is part of excellent client service.

The previous chapter looked at how we communicate and how we can improve our communication skills. This chapter looks specifically at improving people relations through better communication.

## Improving interpersonnel relations

*Customer relations mirror employee relations. The way you treat your employees is the way they will treat your customers.*
Cannie and Caplin, *Keeping Customers for Life*

Good communication in the practice must start with the practice staff; if they do not get on well together then they will certainly not be motivated to help clients.

Signs of an unhappy practice include constant complaining and excessive gossiping among staff, which not only wastes time but stirs trouble too. Staff may grumble and complain overtly, or they may express their feelings more subtly by constantly being late for work, the practice having a high turnover of staff, or by promising new staff members rapidly becoming complacent and doing only the bare minimum.

### Some of the internal problems

#### The practice leader

The *responsibility* for good or bad communication within the practice starts with the practice leader. Communication within the practice creates the attitude which is then conveyed to clients. Thus, a good leader, who is a good communicator, creates a happy practice peopled by happy staff, who work to create happy, satisfied clients. In practices dominated by a bad leader with poor communication skills, staff are typically unhappy, unsure of themselves, and have a cynical and jaded attitude – they are not interested in clients, and the clients sense it.

It is not always easy for a leader to be a good communicator:

> *For example, the director of a residential facility for retarded people was sympathetic to complaints by staff members about their low wages, so he spoke at a meeting with what he thought was forthrightness and concern. He levelled with them by admitting that their jobs would never pay enough to support a family. He also told them they would not be able to advance to higher-paying jobs if they did not have graduate degrees. As their friend, he advised that if they wanted jobs that could lead to more lucrative careers, they would have to find different jobs. The staff did not appreciate their director's candor, because they did not receive his communication as an expression of concern for their welfare coming from a peer. Rather, they heard it as a threat from the boss: 'If you don't like it here, you can jolly well leave.'*
> Deborah Tannen, *You Just Don't Understand*, 1992

Sometimes communication problems have become so severe in a practice that it may be difficult to find solutions.

> *For example, a practice in which I did a consultancy is a prime example of the effect of severe, prolonged communication problems at every level. The principal works half-time in the practice which is resented by all the practice members because:*
>
> - *they don't see him as dedicated to the practice;*
> - *they don't like having to work full time when he does not;*
> - *he is not available when problems arise;*
> - *he uses the Seagull technique of management: flies in every so often, squawks a lot, defecates on several, and flies out again!*

*As a result, they are not happy in their work, they barely co-operate with each other, they give (in his eyes) mediocre service because they don't see why they should really bother with the clients, and take advantage of his 'kindnesses' (such as not clocking-in their working times, not controlling their usage of pet foods and other products for their own pets, etc.). To improve this practice and sort out its many problems, the leader must communicate his wishes and desires more clearly – and listen more attentively to theirs. He needs to give them very clear guidelines about their behaviour, be on site far more and model the behaviour he wants from his staff – or appoint a full-time manager. It is only by constantly and repetitively telling and showing them what he wants, and rewarding them for the right response that their behaviour can change.*

Practice leaders need to be committed to improving communication, and concentrate on developing their own strengths and overcoming their own weaknesses before trying to influence their staff.

### Staff problems

Of course, not all communication problems are the fault of the boss. There are also a number of distinct communication problem areas common to many practices, which are very important:

- lack of job definition;
- unclear expectations;
- lack of team spirit;
- lack of feedback and recognition;
- poor (negative) attitude;
- personality and communication differences.

### ... and some solutions

### Job definition and satisfaction (see also Chapter 6)

Many recent veterinary graduates complain that their actual job bears little resemblance to the job they discussed with their employer before they started. This creates bitterness and frustration which may result in the veterinarian leaving the practice and ultimately leaving the profession. Clear, written job descriptions for *all* staff members (including the practice principals) which the staff member agrees to and signs, plus appropriate training and the know-how to apply that training to their jobs, avoids one of these fundamental sources of dissatisfaction. A job description should not only outline the basic day-to-day routine, but should also include opportunities for career growth and development, implying that additional training over and above that to carry out the basic job must be provided. This applies equally to veterinary surgeons as to their support staff. By creating job satisfaction and a feeling of progress in a position, staff members are more motivated and more likely to stay with a practice (see also Chapter 12).

## Unclear expectations

Not uncommonly in practice, a job is not done, or is not done in a particular way, the effect being to cause anger and disappointment. This situation arises because the *expectations* for the job were not explained clearly enough. It is better to take the risk of seeming pedantic and oversimplistic in your explanation of what you want achieved, and take time over verbal or written instructions than to err on the side of assumption; that is, assume the person knows and understands what you want of them. Many routine procedures can be documented so that there is a standard reference, for example which laboratory to phone for which analyses, how to identify and deal with a telephone emergency, how to clean, label and sterilize surgical instruments,what the practice advises about neutering, and so on.

## Team spirit (see Chapter 6)

For veterinary practice to function most efficiently and effectively, staff need to move away from group mentality and develop team mentality. A practice team is a group of highly communicative, highly motivated veterinarians and support staff from different backgrounds and experiences, who are working towards a common goal. The goal gives the team a framework of shape and direction. Being involved in a team where everyone has equal importance and value provides motivation. Regular team meetings offer an opportunity for everyone to express new ideas and improve work methods, as well as articulate problems and concerns, and offer solutions.

Working as a team does not mean losing individuality, but it does mean enhancing the individual's knowledge and experience by sharing for the common good. Through good communication, this symbiotic sharing benefits the staff, the practice, the clients and the patients.

## Feedback and recognition (see Chapter 7, Motivation, pp. 86–90)

Two of the greatest demotivators are lack of feedback on how a job is performed, and lack of recognition for a job that is well done. Practice principals often believe they give lots of encouragement and positive feedback; their staff tell the opposite. A simple 'thank you' or 'well done' is very rewarding and encouraging. Similarly, where a job is not being well done, correcting in a *positive and constructive* manner helps create the right behaviour.

## Poor (negative) attitude

A negative attitude in an organization is like a malignant cancer; it disfigures and destroys all it touches, it spreads rapidly and is a potent demotivator. A negative attitude expresses itself through people who can only ever see problems, difficulties, faults and obstructions. Sometimes it is an innate character flaw, but more often it is a learnt behaviour that comes from frustration and a feeling of being unable to achieve.

Having a positive attitude means being willing to accept and try new ideas and methods, to look for the good in situations (although being realistic about the bad), and to be constructive and creative rather than destructive.

A positive attitude must come from the top, from the boss. It does not mean the practice need constantly exist in a Pollyanna-like state of euphoria ('I'm so *glad* today!'), but it does mean that it becomes open and receptive rather than closed and disillusioned.

> *It is possible to learn to have a positive attitude. I, along with my veterinary colleagues, was once bluntly told by our appalled new manager, that if we did not change our, then, negative attitudes we would be out of our jobs. Shocked, we did – and were amazed at how different the world suddenly seemed. It was not a place of gloom and despondency where nothing worked and no one co-operated, but a place of optimism, opportunity and friendly people.*

## Personality types and communication differences

Attitudes and styles of working differ according to personality types, so communication can often be confused by individual and personal differences in interpretation of messages. For example, men and women tend to work and communicate in different ways (Lader, 1985; Tannen, 1992) which may be a source of problems, especially as the traditional structure of male principals and female support staff still exists in many practices. An awareness of these differences can help maintain a tolerant and harmonious atmosphere in the practice.

### Improving interpersonnel communication

Some of the solutions to internal communication problems have already been described, but other considerations are:

- spreading information accurately through the practice by having 'division leaders' who are responsible for ensuring that all in their 'division' have received new information, and who also channel information from that 'division' back to the practice leaders;
- circulating written minutes from meetings for everyone to read and sign (this avoids the problem of, 'Oh, I didn't know we'd agreed that . . . ');
- listening to and respecting each others opinions even if you do not necessarily agree with them;
- actively working to collaborate and communicate better together.

## Improving relations with clients

*We depend on our clients, they do not necessarily depend on us.*
Chapter 8, Table 8.3

Veterinary practice is a service industry committed to serving the needs of clients (animal owners and their animals). Practices cannot exist without their clients, and yet increasing competition means clients have more choice than ever before about where to take their animals. Most clients seek good service. Good client service is based on good communication which comes from trust (see Chapter 4, p. 49). The more trust that is developed between staff and clients, the more co-operation and success the clinic will experience.

### Attitude to clients

Staff of veterinary practices are primarily dealing with animal owners, so, first and foremost, they must be 'people people'. A clear definition of the practice's attitude to clients is vital to avoid communication problems (see Chapter 8, p. 111–112).

### Veterinarians as teachers

*Each of us carries around a crippling disadvantage – we know and probably cherish our product. After all, we live with it day in and*

*day out. But that blinds us to why the customer may hate it – or love it. Our customers see the product through an entirely different set of lenses.* **Education is not the answer; listening and adapting is.** (my emphasis)
Tom Peters, Management Consultant

It is very easy for a desire to truly and effectively communicate with clients to become a desire to 'educate' them; that is, 'talk and tell' them. One of the major roles of a veterinarian is as a teacher, but a good teacher does not force his/her views and opinions on his/her pupils and assume they are stupid and ignorant if they do not immediately comprehend what is meant. Veterinarians must be willing to listen to what their clients want and be able to present their message in a way most likely to gain client co-operation and understanding. Clients need to feel *they* are in control, and that *they* are making the decisions concerning their pet's welfare, *not* that they are being pushed into something they do not fully understand.

> *For example, dental disease is a common problem in small breeds of dogs. Veterinarians can educate clients most effectively about prevention of this disease not by showing them calculus-coated teeth and inflamed gums, and assuming the client then feels guilty enough to want to do something about their dog's teeth (but what?): but by devising a whole programme of information and help for the client that will take them in a step-by-step way through dental care, including providing the toothbrushes and other products that can help with dental care, and the continuous support of trained staff to whom the client can refer for help and guidance.*

## Client perception

The client's perception of veterinary practice, and the professional services and products offered are completely different from your own. The client's perception is based on a mixture of personal experience, word-of-mouth information, a bad experience 5 years ago (long and conveniently forgotten by you) and, perhaps, a competitor's recent small act of courtesy. In addition, clients speak a different 'language' from veterinary surgeons and veterinary nurses (just as you speak a different 'language' from nuclear physicists, bankers, or lawyers).

## Satisfying clients' needs

Clients come to veterinary practice because they have needs. Clients' needs may not be the same as their animals' needs; for example the animal requires a vaccination and dental check, the owner may be more concerned about finding a good boarding kennels for the summer.

Dealing with client needs is part of establishing the trust bond. To create a strong bond with the practice, studies have shown that clients want their vet to:

- look and behave like a professional;
- respect that the client's time is valuable too by being on time for appointments;
- show interest in and enthusiasm for them, their pets and their children;
- show affection to the pet;
- handle the pet kindly and not use unnecessary restraint;
- greet them and their pets by name;
- make the client feel like a friend rather than a number by establishing personal contact with them;
- give an accurate estimate of the fees;
- take phone calls from clients requesting information as often as possible.

## First impressions

First impressions are enormously important and you only get one chance to make them! In less than 4 minutes, a person in a new situation makes an, often subconscious, assessment of what they see, hear, smell and touch. These assessments, which are based on a combination of previous experience and intuition, are usually very accurate and can create a strong and lasting impression of a person or place. What does your practice communicate to your clients when they walk in? What do your staff communicate? Do clients get the feeling they matter?

*Imagine the difference in impression two clients would have if the first one walked into a practice that is spotlessly clean, attractively decorated, the staff are welcoming and friendly, and the veterinarian greets them by name, compared to the scene facing the second client who walks in behind a case of haemorraghic diarrhoea where there are stinking, bloody pools of faeces on the floor, the staff are harrassed, and the veterinarian is so busy the client is forced to wait half an hour. Of course, situations like this can occur in the best practices, but it is important to strive to continually keep the practice as you want every client to see it. First impressions are enormously important!*

Using the same four senses, you make a snapshot analysis of a client when you first meet them which then influences your attitude towards them. You assess their apparent financial standing, their age, general health and attitude. You assess the feelings they show for their pet through physical and verbal contact. Your first impression can have a profound effect on, for example, the services and standard of care you think they can afford and the level of care they would like for their pet.

Of course, while you are assessing your clients, they are assessing you! What do you communicate to your clients in those first 4 minutes? Do you communicate professionalism and competence by looking smart and efficient, or do you communicate disinterest and lack of care? Your professional appearance is enormously important because not only is it the way clients initially assess you but it can affect all future relations between you.

## Some general comments

When you talk to a client you are usually trying to persuade them of the value of your ideas for the care and treatment of their pet: you are literally 'selling' yourself and your concepts to them. For them to 'buy' they must believe and trust you. This trust comes through not only what you say and how you say it, but in having a confident, friendly, and reassuring manner. This is demonstrated by maintaining at least 60% eye contact (would you trust anyone who cannot meet your eye?), gestures such as stroking the pet as you talk, and so on.

Do not forget to talk to the pet too – although read their body language signals with care to avoid being bitten or scratched! Most pets will give you plenty of indication that they will not welcome your advances. Owners bring their pets to you because you are the expert in animal care, and they assume you like animals too. The vet who doesn't stroke their pet, or, at least, say hello to it, and jumps away if the pet attempts to sniff them will soon get a reputation for not being able to handle animals and therefore not being a very good vet.

When speaking to clients, or writing instructions or handouts, avoid scientific jargon. Do not rush through explanations as this may give them a feeling of being 'brushed off'. It may be the hundredth time you have explained about the importance of regular vaccination today, but it is the first time that *this* client has heard it. Don't assume a superior manner – client relations are not improved if they feel 'put down'.

## Improving communication in the reception area

The reception area is the first area the client sees in the practice. It is ideal for communicating some of the basic values of the practice, such as:

- *We care about our clients* – make the area as attractive, comfortable and welcoming as possible.
- *We are a professional team* – photograph boards with the staff, their qualifications (and their pets) tell clients who works here.
- *We give top animal health care* – posters, and product displays inform clients about preventive health care in the practice; and so on.

## The role of the receptionist in communication

The receptionist is one of the key people in the practice and is usually the first person the client meets and speaks to. A receptionist's job is far more than simply managing the front desk and the telephone; a receptionist communicates the practice's professional image to the client by manner, appearance and attitude. It is especially important to hire a receptionist who is interested in people and their animals.

## Improving communication in the consulting room

> *Your exam room demeanour can bond clients to your practice – or chase them away ... (Improving communication in the exam room) ... is a challenge well worth the effort, as effective communication can be not only fun, but supremely rewarding to you and your cash flow.*
> R. Clark, Veterinary Practice Management Consultant

The consulting room offers many opportunities over and above discussions of medical and surgical treatment to communicate the values of the practice to your clients (see Table 5.1).

Improve communication by attention to detail:

- take a personal interest in each case;
- get the sex of the pet right;
- call pet and owner by their right names;

**Table 5.1** *More effective consulting room communication*

- Introduce yourself
- Touch and talk to the pet
- Present yourself as a professional
- Be an active listener and ask good questions
- Talk about the *benefits* of treatment/professional products/drugs,. etc.
- Use visual information
- Give educational handouts
- Compliment the client
- Explain the best treatment options first
- Make sure you've answered all of the client's questions

- read the records and be informed about the case before seeing the pet;
- always use an assistant to restrain the pet;
- ensure the room is scrupulously clean and odour free;
- provide a chair for the owner to sit on.

### Managing the difficult client

*You can please some of the people all of the time, but you cannot please all of the people all of the time.*
Anon

Working in practice, you are required to be much more than just 'good with animals'; you are aiming to create and maintain a high level of goodwill with your colleagues and clients. However, you deal with a cross-section of the community daily, and it is inevitable that some clients will not be satisfied with the job you have done. Studies show that 70% of clients with grievances will stay with the practice if efforts are made to remedy their complaint; 95% will stay if their complaint is rectified on the spot.

The main sources of irritation to clients are:

- *Waiting too long to see the vet* – clients' time is valuable too.
- *Not receiving an accurate estimate of the bill* – for procedures over a certain value (say £250) give clients a written quotation which they sign. Update clients, and gain their consent if actual costs are going to exceed the original estimate.
- *That the vet/staff handled the pet roughly* – especially important when the pet is being euthanased. Teach staff how to handle pets confidently and kindly, and explain to clients what you are doing and why.

Anticipating these problems and formulating methods for resolving them *before they arise* can help prevent unpleasant scenes occurring.

> *For example, as a young graduate, I once grossly underestimated the costs of surgery to remove a foreign body from a dog who had eaten a sheepskin rug. The owner refused to pay the final, much higher fee, saying he would have had the dog put down if he had realized how much it was going to cost. My boss intervened and decided to accept payment based on the original quotation, and although the practice lost money on that occasion – I certainly didn't made the same mistake again! The practice, however, lost the client and this is not the best way – in business terms – to learn by experience.*

Some clients are only rude to support staff and are perfectly civilized with the veterinarians. The receptionist is frequently in the front line for abuse from clients and has to bear the brunt of their aggression and anger. Clients should be shown that everybody in the practice is an equally valued team member, and staff should be empowered to resolve problems. If they are unable to do so, then the complainant should be referred to the practice manager.

## Dealing with grief

Euthanasia of a pet is probably the most emotionally loaded and stressful procedure a veterinary surgeon performs. It is also, in the client's eyes, more memorable for being performed well – or badly – than all the heroic surgery or medical procedures their pet may have undergone.

A grief-stricken client may be almost hysterical with misery or may be highly abusive. Either way, they can be a disturbing and traumatic category of people to deal with. The distress may be due to a sudden and unexpected death or from a recent decision to euthanase a chronically ill pet. It can also be complicated by previous experiences of death of loved family members.

> *For example, an elderly lady agreed to euthanasia of her old and ill labrador a week before Christmas. She broke down in floods of tears, and explained to me between sobs that her husband had died a year ago, her beloved son-in-law six months later, and now her only remaining link to them was dead too. And only now could she grieve; before she'd had to concentrate so hard on keeping a "stiff upper lip", being in control and not breaking down in front of family and freinds.*

Grief passes through a number of stages which are a normal part of the grieving process. They include disbelief and shock, anger, guilt, depression and acceptance of the death (Kübler-Ross, 1970) and the grieving person can be in any of them. Be prepared to be patient, empathetic and understanding – and tolerant if the client is abusive. Ensure your support staff can handle the situation sensitively. Men in particular can be very shocked at the amount of grief they feel, and may think you are secretly laughing at their tears. Choose your words carefully. Phrases such as, 'Well, you can always get another dog,' or 'But Fluffy was only an ordinary cat' are grossly insensitive but unfortunately are still heard in veterinary clinics. Try to be impartial about the client's decision too, even if you would not have made the same decision.

Preparing the owner beforehand for what is involved with a voluntary euthanasia, and allowing them a quiet room where they can cry privately rather than leaving them waiting in a busy reception area help make the euthanasia less traumatic. The option for a home euthanasia is often very welcome, reducing the stress for the pet and owner alike. It is very important to take time over the procedure and, where you know the owner and pet well, phone or send a handwritten card a few days later expressing your condolences. For many people, losing a pet is like losing a human friend – but society does not allow them to mourn in the same way. Performing a euthanasia, for whatever reason, is a very sensitive time: veterinarians are not taught now to manage grief, either the clients' or their own. Treat the situation with great care. It is one of the most likely situations to be reported to the RCVS if handled badly.

### External lecturing

Another way in which veterinarians communicate with clients – who may be animal owners or colleagues with referral cases – is through lectures and presentations. There is an art to giving a good presentation, and while it is not possible to describe it in detail here you *can* improve your presentation technique by attention to the following points:

- identify your audience clearly, for example their technical knowledge, age, interests;
- what message are you conveying? Is this a technical presentation to colleagues? A marketing presentation about herd health for farmers? Information about correct nutrition for breeders?;
- identify size of audience – a slide presentation is ideal for a large group but may be too formal for a group of six, say;

- prepare your presentation carefully, and practice it out loud so that you can give it fluently;
- be prepared to answer questions;
- *Keep it short*: a maximum concentration span is 45 minutes. For a successful presentation, do not exceed this.

## ■ **Summary** ■

1 Good communication with clients starts with good inter-personnel communication.

2 Common reasons for bad staff communication include poor leadership, lack of team spirit, and a negative attitude.

3 Client relations can be improved by treating them as individuals, paying attention to detail, and taking time to explain things to them.

# 6 Employing Professional and Support Staff: Creating a Team

*All organizations depend for their success on people . . .*

Roger Oldcorn, Management Consultant

VETERINARY practices compete in two marketplaces: they compete for clients who *provide* the business, and they compete for staff who *are* the business. Systems and strategies are present in most veterinary practices to a greater or lesser extent to attract clients, but how many practices think seriously about recruiting the right staff? What are the parameters needed to select the right staff? How are staff encouraged to work really effectively?

The next two chapters look at how to make the most of your staff. In this chapter, staff recruitment and converting staff into a more effective unit or team is discussed. Chapter 7 outlines the role of the practice leader in gaining optimal personal and team performance through delegation, empowerment, motivation and performance asessment.

## Recruiting staff

Your staff are critical to the success of your practice, so it is worth taking time and effort with their selection. What are you seeking from them? Knowledge? Skills (experience)? Attitude? Professional *knowledge* can be codified and easily shared; professional *skills*, such as winning the trust and confidence of animal owners, and making the myriad judgemental decisions as to how each case should be handled, although highly personalized, can be developed with practice. *Attitude*, however, is the method by which these attributes are shared with clients. To create a happy, healthy practice, you need to hire attitude.

The primary role of both professional and support staff is to create trust with people, both to ensure a harmonious work relationship with colleagues, and to develop a friendly and productive business relationship with clients. Staff therefore need to be people-oriented – that is, interested in and concerned to help people and their animals. And they need to be good communicators, both within the practice and with clients. They also need to be positive, forward thinking and open to new ideas.

There are a number of stages to the recruiting process. I recommend taking time over each stage, planning carefully, and involving other staff members in your decisions. The method outlined below is not fool-proof, but it should help you find the best people available for your practice.

## Define the job

What, exactly, is the job you wish done? What characteristics are you looking for in your candidate? It is *not* enough to simply employ a 'veterinary surgeon' or 'receptionist'. Discuss what is needed with other members of staff, and draw up a detailed job description.

It may seem pedantic to do this – surely a veterinary surgeon/nurse/ receptionist knows what they are expected to do in a practice! – but preparing a job description has numerous advantages:

- It clarifies exactly what the practice needs – and can afford.
- It clarifies what the job truly entails for the successful candidate.
- It provides a basis for measurable performance parameters (see Chapter 7).
- It reduces the potential for misunderstandings (see Chapter 5, p. 57).

It is important to clarify expectations, both of what you want from your successful candidate, and of what they expect to receive from the job in the way of salary, further training, continuing education, and so on. Many staff members end up frustrated and disappointed because 'promises' made at the interview never materialize.

> *For example, are you seeking a veterinarian with specialist skills in surgery or medicine, or an untrained graduate? If the latter, how much time are you prepared to spend training and helping them to get them up to speed? What sort of personality are you seeking to fit into your practice team and to relate to clients? What are the hours and conditions he/she is expected to work? What proportion of time will be spent on clinical duties? Surgical duties? Farm visits? What is the future for this veterinarian in your practice?*

The specific job description also has to link with the practice policies on, for example, recommending and selling general health care products such as pet foods, behaviour towards clients, charging policies and so on. There are also certain points which must be included in any Contract of Employment (see Table 6.1).

A basic job description for a veterinary nurse working in the consulting area in a large practice could be:

- assisting the consulting veterinarian(s);
- maintaining a friendly, helpful attitude to clients;
- weighing every pet before a consultation;
- taking X-rays, blood tests, urine samples, etc. as requested and dealing with them as appropriate;

**Table 6.1** *Fifteen essential points in a contract of employment*

1  The full names of all the parties concerned, i.e. the employer and employee.
2  Date of commencement of employment and of continuous employment.
3  Method of calculating salary (or scale or rate of remuneration), and when the salary will be paid (e.g. weekly, monthly).
4  Terms and conditions that exist relating to hours of work or normal working hours.
5  Terms and conditions that exist relating to holiday entitlement such as public holidays and holiday pay. This must be given in sufficient detail to enable calculation of ongoing holiday entitlement and entitlement accruing at termination.
6  Terms and conditions relating to sick leave including sick pay provision.
7  Terms and conditions relating to pensions.
8  Length of termination notice required from either side.
9  Job description and/or job title.
10  The place of work for the employee, or a statement with the employer's address stating that the employee must work at several locations.
11  For temporary employment, the period for which the employment will continue; for fixed-term contract, the date when that contract expires.
12  Details of the practice's disciplinary procedure, including appeals.
13  Details of the practice's grievance procedure including appeals.
14  Any collective agreements that directly affect the terms and conditions of employment including, where the employer is not a party, the parties to such agreements.
15  (Not usually applicable to general practice) If the employee is required to work outside the UK for more than 1 month, the period of work outside the UK, the currency in which he is to be paid, any additional payments and benefits to be provided, and any terms relating to the employee's return to the UK.

■ ensuring clients receive the medicines, health care products, etc. that have been prescribed or recommended, and that they understand how to use them;

■ ensuring clients are properly billed for procedures;

■ ensuring the consulting area is always clean, that uniforms are clean, etc.;

■ ensuring the consulting rooms are always properly stocked with drugs and disposables.

## What pay and conditions can we offer?

*If you pays peanuts, you gets monkeys.*
Anon

Many veterinary assistants are, unfortunately, still grossly underpaid. This is a reflection both of the attitude of low self-worth still prevalent within the profession, and of the lack of career structure available. What, for example, should you pay the 'mature, experienced assistant'? To attract high calibre veterinarians, practices should strive to offer significantly better and different salary packages – based on the veterinarian fulfilling defined expectations of productivity.

As the ability of your practice to recruit and pay for the best of employees is a direct function of your profitability, to pay more than the average rate the practice must ensure that sufficient additional revenue is generated. It is important that employees understand that they are largely responsible for generating their own income through correct charging for services performed, and from attracting new clients.

Many practices hire untrained, unskilled support staff because they are cheap. In most cases this actually proves to be more expensive. The only factor binding them to the job is the wage – if they can earn better elsewhere, they will go elsewhere. In the long run, this wastes more time (and money) seeking and training new staff than is saved by hiring cheap labour.

## Advertising the position

Advertising is the usual way to seek potential applicants, and advertisements should be short, clear and request a written curriculum vitae/ resume be sent with a letter of application for the position. Good staff may also be found by word of mouth and 'head-hunting', that is, identifying someone by their skills and abilities and enticing them to join your practice. However, be careful not to infringe the Equal Opportunity regulations.

### Review of applications

Information from the letter and CV sent in by the applicant eliminates many applicants early on. For those in whom you are interested, check their references. An informal phone-call to a former employer may give a lot more information about the true value of a candidate than is apparent from their CV, and past performance can give a clear prediction of future performance. (However, this can be a delicate situation as although the present employer may be the best reference, he or she may not yet be aware of the person's application.)

> 'Headhunted' staff members should still go through all the interview process (see below) to ensure they really are right for the practice. A practice principal I know was delighted when he successfully 'headhunted' the apparently perfect veterinary surgeon; she was medically and surgically very competent, as well as having an excellent manner with clients. However, within a few months, the story was very different. He was not aware of her chronic physical and mental health problems, which included severe backache and depression, and which had a marked effect on her ability to work. Had this principal investigated her past records more carefully, he might have avoided hiring someone who ultimately turned out to be unable to perform her job satisfactorily and had to have her contract terminated.

### Planning for interview

An interview is like a conversation with a purpose, the purpose being to find out how truly suited the applicant is for the job in question. An interview requires careful planning. What do you need to know about the applicant?

Asking open-ended questions will generally give far more information than closed questions that require a yes/no answer. For example, ask the applicant to say what they like and dislike about their present job. What is their greatest achievement so far (professionally or personally)? What would they like to be doing 5 years from now?

An interview is not only to examine an applicant with a view to their suitability, but also to inform the applicant about the practice and present it in a favourable, but truthful!, light so that the applicant is attracted to the practice.

Arrange the interview by appointment and make sure the applicant has a contact name and number to ring if he/she has to change the arrangement. Explain the practice policy on providing lunch/paying for travel/overnight accommodation/etc.

## Conducting the interview

The interview should be planned to elicit information from the applicant which will enable his or her experience, qualifications and personal qualities to be measured against the requirements set out in the job specification. Have at least two people involved in the interview to get different impressions of the candidate.

When interviewing, set the applicant at ease by being friendly and welcoming and explain how you are going to conduct the interview. Briefly explain a little about the job and the practice. It is not necessary to spend a long time over this, especially if you are unsure how suitable the applicant is – you can always take time later to fill in the details. Get the applicant to provide a brief autobiographical account of his/her working life so far by asking about their current job. What are their plans for the future? Try to get an impression of their attitude as well as their abilities; for example ask them about the worst thing they've done – and the best thing. Probing questions that will reveal the applicant's true feelings can also be very helpful, for example ask a potential receptionist questions such as:

- What would you do if a pet urinates in the reception area?
- How would you handle a client who is rude to you at the reception desk?
- If you own a pet, what role does it play in your family?
- What do you feel about pet euthanasia?

It is important to identify strong opinions or attitudes before offering a job to avoid later surprises and frustrations for both parties (see Table 6.2).

Finally, allow time at the end of the interview for further questions before showing the applicant around the practice and introducing him/her to key members of staff. Ask them their opinions of the applicant afterwards.

*A veterinary surgeon applied for the position of assistant in the practice I was working in. She arrived for the interview with the practice principal with her hair tied back in a rubber-band, wearing an old skirt and blouse, open-toed sandals which showed a large hole in the toe of her tights, and with dirty fingernails. Needless to say, although she was pleasant to talk to, none of the staff was impressed with her 'professional appearance (attitude)' and she was not hired.*

**Table 6.2** *Do's and Dont's of interviewing*

**Do:**
- Have a clear description of the job for which the applicant is being interviewed
- Plan the interview
- Encourage the applicant to talk
- Establish an easy and informal relationship
- Follow the interview plan and cover all that you had planned
- Probe deeper as necessary
- Analyse career and interests (both personal and professional) to reveal strengths, weaknesses and patterns of behaviour
- Maintain control over the direction and time taken by the interview
- Consider the applicant as a whole – balance the good and the bad in relation to the requirements of the job

**Don't:**
- Start the interview unprepared
- Go too quickly into difficult, demanding questions
- Ask leading questions
- Jump to conclusions on inadequate evidence
- Pay too much attention to particular strengths and weaknesses in isolation
- Allow the applicant to gloss over important facts
- Talk too much yourself

### Evaluate the interview

Does the applicant measure up to the standards you have set? No one will be the 'perfect fit' – they are always 'almost fits', but some people will fit a lot better than others.

### Final selection

Decisions about people are time-consuming, but should not be hurried. Don't make too many compromises. It is important to find the right person. Interview potential candidates a second time if necessary. If none of the applicants is really what you want, go back to the beginning and start again. Review your advertisement – is it attracting the right sort of applicants? Do you need to change it? It may be frustrating to start again, but it will be much more beneficial for everyone in the long run.

## Unsuitable staff

Sometimes mistakes are made and staff are found to be so unsuitable that it is felt necessary to remove them from the practice. Every employer should be fully aware of the strict regulations governing termination of a contract. The *BVA Guide to an Agreement Between Principals and Assistants* and *BVA Guide to Contracts* provide useful summaries, and the most current edition of the booklet detailing the *Employment Protection Act* should also be referred to (available from Her Majesty's Stationery Office).

Some key points about dismissal are that a person cannot be given less than 1 week's notice (unless they have been employed in full-time work for less than 1 month), and usually require at least a strict verbal and preferably a written warning to avoid a charge of unfair dismissal. Gross misconduct, such as dishonesty, gross neglect and breach of safety rules, wilful refusal to follow lawful and reasonable instruction, and persistent drunkenness, may justify summary dismissal but there is usually time and justification for a warning before action.

## ■ Conducting an exit interview

Staff represent an investment of time, money and effort. It can be frustrating and disappointing for a practice if they resign. Exit interviews provide an opportunity for a candid review of the factors that have brought about their resignation and may, sometimes, be a chance to reverse their decision. An exit interview can give valuable insights into problems within the practice – and provide an opportunity to do something about them.

Ideally, the interview should not be conducted by the person's immediate boss or supervisor, and should preferably be performed off the premises or even over the telephone. The aim is to gain information in a relaxed, informal way rather than to interrogate the person. Useful questions to ask include:

- Would you come back?
- What did you learn from working here?
- Was the job description you received accurate?
- If not, why not?
- Do you feel you received adequate training/support/etc. to be able to conduct your job well?
- Were you treated fairly?
- If not, where was the treatment lacking?
- What did you like most about working here?
- What did you like least?
- What would you change about your job?
- What was your relationship like with other practice members/ specific practice members (e.g. the boss, the manager, the head nurse)?

■ How could the practice – or individuals within the practice – do a better job to help and support your position in future?

If there is time, it may be advisable to ask the person leaving to prepare written answers to these questions so that their answers are more focused, and therefore of more use to you. Thank them for their participation. And use the information they give you!

## ■■■■ Creating a practice team

*No one individual has all the necessary skills to provide a complete service for all clients, but by combining all staff skills . . . (veterinarian, nurse and receptionist) . . . the needs of the client, patient and practice are met.*
Dennis McCurnin, Veterinary Management Consultant

The staff of veterinary practices traditionally function as groups rather than teams. Groups tend to live day-by-day, completing only those aspects of their jobs that are necessary, and typically suffer from lack of communication and low motivation.

Teams are quite different. A team is defined as: *a highly communicative group of individuals with different background skills and abilities, who have a common purpose, and who work together to achieve clearly defined goals.* They are characterized by:

■ purpose;
■ good relationships based on excellent communication;
■ high levels of performance from all team members;
■ flexibility and imagination;
■ confidence and high morale;
■ recognition and appreciation of each other.

Converting a group to a team is not easy. Veterinarians, for example, are not taught to be interdependent – they learn to function as isolated, independent-thinking individuals. (It is interesting to note, however, that most veterinarians appreciate support from colleagues, which is the major reason for choosing to work in multi-vet practices.) Team members do not have to be all 'jolly hockey-sticks' together. They do not even have to get on particularly well – but they have to be able to accomplish things together.

There are many advantages to learning to think and behave like a team. A good team:

- Collaborates and co-operates to create a symbiotic relationship – the total result is greater than the sum of the parts.
- Works for common goals, staff are more involved and have better 'ownership' of the practice, which makes them more committed and productive.
- Offers improved medical care for patients: *'The health care system of the future will place more emphasis on the decision-making abilities of a team of individuals working together – a team that should include the . . . (client-owner) . . .'* (I.S. Udvarhelyi, Vice President, Prudential Insurance Co, 1994).
- Offers improved practice productivity and profitability.
- Offers opportunities for improved personal growth and development.

So, how do you go about converting your staff-group into a team?

### The team leader

Team building is a matter of establishing mutual trust and confidence among the group of people working for you. Your aim, as practice principal and team leader, is to create a feeling of interdependence, a feeling of shared responsibility for getting results.

There are six areas a leader can concentrate on to start the conversion of a group to a team:

- Create the right environment in which to establish a team through having a positive, cheerful working attitude that encourages communication and participation.
- Identify at a very early stage the common mission or purpose of the team (see Chapter 2, p. 23 for writing a practice mission; and Chapter 3, p. 33 for writing a personal mission). To stimulate and motivate the participants, creating the mission should be a collective decision-making process.
- Encourage participation in agreeing objectives and targets and establish common goals collectively.
- Rotate jobs within the team, where feasible, to get members to identify with the team as a whole rather than just the job.
- Ensure communications flow freely.
- Get people acting in the way that you want by constantly modelling that behaviour, and rewarding them for responding. Gradually they'll come to believe in what they're doing.

A word of caution. Some people just aren't 'team types' – they are better as 'solo performers'. Hackman (1994) writes:

> *These are people who just don't have the skills to work construc-*
> *tively in teams – and who are unable or unwilling to acquire those*
> *skills . . . There are only three ways to deal with them when teams*
> *are formed. One, keep them at a safe distance from the teams so*
> *they can do no damage . . . Two, go ahead and put them on teams*
> *. . . (under) . . . strong leaders . . . and hope for the best . . . (Three)*
> *. . . harvest the contributions of (these) talented people . . . in a way*
> *that does not put the team itself at risk.*

Faced with this situation in your practice, you will have to decide if a non-team person's abilities are so valuable that the practice needs them at all costs, or whether the team's development would be better off without them.

## Stages of team development

Groups become effective teams in stages (Blanchard *et al.*, 1993) which can take a variable amount of time.

### Stage 1: Orientation
New team members feel eager, have high expectations, some anxiety, and there is a certain amount of jostling for position.

### Stage 2: Dissatisfaction
Many groups never progress beyond this highly unproductive stage which is characterized by feelings of dissatisfaction, frustration, incompetence and confusion. There is often a negative feeling towards the team leader and the group may feel it is not worth progressing. Just knowing that this awkward stage exists and is inevitable can help a good leader guide the team on to the next stage.

### Stage 3: Resolution
Harmony, trust, support and respect develops as the polarities and animosities between members start to resolve. Self-esteem and confidence come back. Members use a team language and begin to share responsibility and control.

### Stage 4: Production

Team members now collaborate enthusiastically together, feel very positive about team success and perform at a high level.

Good leadership drives the group forward through the different stages by close observation of the way the individual team members *function together*. This involves looking at how the individuals communicate with each other and how much they participate, the degree of conflict within the group, its ability to make decisions and so on.

## Teaching the team to be a team

### Developing key characteristics

Four key characteristics of a team are commitment, co-operation, communication and contribution. These are learned characteristics which enable the team to become creative, imaginative – and more effective.

Commitment comes from participation in decision making and the feeling that 'my opinion is of value'. But commitment must also be shown by the practice leader. A leader who is not committed – or is not seen to be committed – cannot expect commitment from his or her staff.

> *This apparent lack of commitment from the practice principal is a common reason why teams fail in practice. Principals often throw in ideas, tell the 'team' to get on with them, then take no further interest in them. Another frequent scenario is practice principals who regularly disappear for their game of golf, leaving the 'team' to carry on without them. Although I am not suggesting that principals should have to work 24 hours a day, they have to be able to portray commitment. They have to model the behaviour they want from their staff.*

Co-operation arises from the shared sense of purpose and mutual gain that the practice mission should give. Good communication is vital and can be improved by facing and dealing with controversy, avoiding secrets, and striving to be as open as possible with all team members.

Contribution by all team members to a team is essential. Lack of contribution is demoralizing for those who do contribute – they feel they carry the weight of the team. It may also be reflected to the client in higher overheads – someone has to pay for the non-productive team member.

## Positive attitude

The importance of a positive attitude in a practice team cannot be over-stressed. A positive team concentrates on the strengths and possibilities in a situation rather than the weaknesses and faults.

A positive attitude can be fostered by teaching team members to present information in a positive manner ('I see *x* as a problem, but think a solution could be . . .') and using effective feedback rather than 'constructive criticism'; that is, attack the problem, not the person. Encouraging innovation and innovative ideas stimulates a positive attitude; it shows that you recognize that limiting the practice to the current ideas within the profession is not the way forward. Again, your behaviour is crucial; modelling a positive attitude is the most important thing you can do to help your team's attitude.

## Motivation

Motivation comes from how the practice rewards behaviour. For example:

- Do staff who work long hours and look busy get rewarded against those who get results?
- Are demands made for quality work, but no guidelines given as to how to achieve quality?
- Are staff frightened to be different and yet the boss always complains about lack of initiative?
- Is team work demanded, but one team member played off against another?

The definition of a team is that its members are motivated. How you can motivate your team is discussed in Chapter 7.

## Team meetings

Team meetings are an essential activity for a healthy team. Meetings can include everything from a quick chat in the corridor to a formal meeting of all staff in the practice. They should be an extremely effective way of improving communication in a practice, but all too often they are total time-wasters.

Meetings are called for a variety of reasons:

- *Information dissemination:* for example, new information about a vaccine.
- *Problem-solving meetings:* for example, there is a problem with the telephone service that needs a solution.

- *creative-thinking meetings:* for example, how can we inform clients about our new dental health programmme?
- *Miscellaneous*.

Meetings can be made inspiring, stimulating and successful by sticking to the following guidelines:

- Keep them short – maximum 1 hour.
- Start and end on time.
- Have a predetermined agenda (see below) and stick to it.
- Control the meeting by ensuring members do not dominate the meeting and that everyone has a chance to contribute.
- Only involve those who are necessary but keep everyone informed of the outcomes.
- Rotate chairmanship of the meeting so that everyone in the practice has the opportunity to organize and chair meetings.
- Make sure all the relevant information (facts, figures) is available – if necessary prepare handouts.
- Involve everyone in the meeting by asking for their contributions
- Ensure people stick to the subject under discussion and that their remarks are relevant.
- Use written minutes which are circulated to and signed by all members of the practice.

## Meeting agenda

Everyone in the practice should have the opportunity to contribute to forming the agenda; for example, by having a sheet of paper in the staff room where suggestions can be written for topics for discussion. The chairperson should then select the five or six issues that can be included in the meeting.

In addition, every agenda should include:

- *Achievements and mistakes:* ask the team to briefly outline achievements and mistakes since the last meeting. This gives the opportunity to praise successes and assess errors.
- *Follow up* from the last meeting on what was decided. Has everyone done what they promised they would do?
- *Devise the new action plan* for the week/month. This is not an opportunity for complaints, but for positive suggestions and ways of improving systems in the practice to be put forward.
- *Rewards and recognition:* praise and reward those who have done a good job. Make sure everybody gets some sort of recognition.

- *Professional development:* ask a team member or invite a speaker in to share some interesting information. It could be on a new surgical technique, a new diagnostic test, or a better way to answer the telephone. Videos and audiotapes can also be useful in this context.
- *General announcements* – to save time these can be typed up before- hand and distributed. Comments can be invited.

## Why teams fail

Teams fail for a variety of reasons. The most common is that team members don't know what they are supposed to be doing – they do not have a clear understanding of the practice goals and their role in working for them.

Other problems are that the team member doesn't know how to do what he is expected to, or that he can't do it. In the former case more time may be needed to better explain expectations and for training; in the latter, the selection process may be wrong.

> *For example, a goal for the team might be to increase client numbers by 3% over the next 3 months. There would have to be discussion and agreement among the team members to achieve this goal otherwise nothing will come of it.*
>
> *Asking a veterinarian who has primarily worked with cattle and cattle farmers, to develop a full-service feline speciality in the practice would probably reflect the wrong selection process. It is not that they could not do it, it is just that they probably have not the experience (or interest or sensitivity to handle other types of clients) to do the job well.*

Sometimes teams fail because members simply won't co-operate – they refuse to do what is asked of them. Insubordination can arise from not understanding what is being asked of them, or not agreeing with it. It can usually be overcome by giving the team member clear reasons for doing what is requested of them, giving them plenty of access to supporting information, and encouraging them by rewarding the right behaviour – with a reward of value to the person in question. The importance of constantly modelling the right behaviour yourself cannot be overstressed.

*A common example of team-insubordination that I have come*

*across is veterinarians refusing to promote nutrition for healthy pets in their practices because they associate it with becoming 'pet food salespeople'. They are being insubordinate to the support staff who already see the advantages of selling nutrition backed with a veterinary recommendation for healthy pets. Given time and plenty of supportive information, veterinarians eventually accept the benefits of promoting healthy nutrition and realize their image of becoming pet-food salespeople is mistaken.They also reap the rewards of knowing they are doing a better job in disease prevention and health maintenance for pets, and enhance practice income.*

A staff member who persists in not co-operating may be better out of the practice.

## ◼︎ Levels of staffing

*The more people are together, the more time their sheer interaction will take, the less will be available for them to work, accomplish and get results.*
Peter Drucker, Senior Management Consultant

Overstaffing – that is, employing too many people for the real work available – is a common problem. Too many people simply get in each other's way. The exponential increase in the number of possible staff interactions that occurs also increases the potential for time-wasting, boredom, and mischief-making. People become an impediment to performance.

In a lean organization, people have room to move without colliding with one another and can do their work without having to explain it all the time. They may have to work harder, but most people respond to a little 'stretching'.

*Under*staffing creates work problems too. Constantly being stressed and overworked is as detrimental, in the long run, as boredom.

It can be very difficult to get the perfect balance of staff in practice where there are daily, monthly and even yearly variations in the volume of work to be done. Training and motivating existing staff to be more effective, using part-time staff for peak periods, and hiring specialist or locum help as needed, are all methods of reducing the problems from under- and overstaffing. The *ratio* of staff is discussed in Chapter 7, pp. 96–98.

# Conclusion

*In the next decade and beyond, the ability to attract, develop, retain and deploy staff will be the single biggest determinant of a professional service firm's competitive success.*
David Maister, Business Management Consultant

# Summary

1   Good staff are critical for practice success.

2   Having good staff starts with hiring them.

3   Staff are most effective when working as a team.

# 7 Effective Staff Management: Putting Leadership Skills into Action

*Management . . . needs concrete, tangible, clear practices. These practices must stress building on strength rather than weakness. They must motivate excellence.*

Peter Drucker, Management Consultant

PERFORMANCE assessment is a method of getting results through people; it measures the individual and/or team achievement of goals or tasks defined by the practice. For most veterinary principals, performance appraisal of staff is a whole new concept, but is integral to improving the efficacy of practice members.

Performance results are the principal's responsibility and there are four primary strategies a principal can use to stimulate performance:

- motivation;
- performance assessment;
- delegation;
- empowerment.

This chapter suggests ways to use these techniques effectively to achieve top performance from a veterinary team.

## Motivation

*People who feel good about themselves produce good results.*
Blanchard and Johnson, *The One Minute Manager*, 1982

Motivation is *the degree of commitment to a course of action and is measured by the effort put into the action*. It is a highly complex issue, so what motivates one individual may have little effect on another, and the effect of removing a demotivator may not always be to motivate; for example a pay cut is usually a demotivator, but a large pay rise may not stimulate harder or better work (see Table 7.1).

Most staff are motivated when they first join a practice and are willing and interested to help clients who, of course, provide the business. However, staff often lose that motivation over time and become less productive. The role of the practice manager (principal/leader) is to build up and maintain high levels of motivation which simultaneously builds staff effectiveness.

## Theories of motivation

There are many theories of motivation, all based on satisfying needs such as material requirements (food, drink, shelter, money), social and esteem needs, and growth needs (self-development and self-actualization). However, research on motivation carried out within factories and offices over the last 50 years has failed to produce convincing evidence that satisfaction of these needs *consistently* leads to good performance. *Satisfaction alone* is not a motivator; effort depends on the *rewards* people expect to get. This, in turn, depends on the value of the reward to the individual and the likelihood of getting that reward (which is based on how

**Table 7.1** *Understanding motivation*

- *Be motivated to motivate others* – a leader must be motivated to motivate his or her team
- *Motivation requires a goal* – it is impossible for an individual or a team to be motivated without a goal
- *Motivation once established does not last* – motivation is like blowing up a balloon – if you don't tie a knot in the inlet, the air will come out again. Motivation is a constant, ongoing process
- *Motivation requires recognition* – people strive harder for recognition than almost anything else in life. Reward and praise success
- *Participation motivates* – feeling they are part of something gives people a higher level of motivation
- *Personal progression motivates* – going forward, whether in a personal or business situation, motivates people to try harder
- *Challenge only motivates if you can win* – the greater the chance of winning, the greater the effort applied
- *Everybody has a motivational fuse* – a good leader provides the light that sparks it
- *Group belonging motivates* – the smaller the unit, the greater the loyalty, motivation and effort given to the group

difficult the job is seen to be and the amount of effort involved). The higher the value of the reward and the probability of receiving it, the greater the effort that will be made in that situation.

Other factors that affect motivation are:

- *Ability* – the individual's intelligence, skills and know-how.
- *Perceptions about the job* – the individual's interpretation of the job (which should be the same as the organization's).
- *Influence of other people* – peer and group pressures are important as they affect social and esteem needs.
- *The job itself* – the extent to which the work itself gives people an opportunity for achievement, responsibility and satisfaction.

## The problem of motivation in veterinary practice

Motivation in veterinary practice is increasingly a problem for veterinary leaders, often as a reflection of a demotivated leader: an unmotivated person cannot motivate others. Demotivation is signalled by a cynical and negative attitude, unwillingness to do anything let alone try something new, and a marked drop in productivity.

Some of the most important reasons veterinarians become demotivated are:

- Veterinarians are often described as 'Type A' people – highly driven, highly self-critical and highly insecure. This somewhat neurotic combination of attributes, although contributing on the one hand to the brilliance and commitment shown by veterinarians can, on the other, be a crippling demotivator through over-harsh judgement of self.
- There is no career structure for veterinarians. What does a veterinarian do after 5, 10, 15 years in practice? Veterinarians need goals to work towards to give themselves direction and purpose. If these are lacking – which, in business, would often be recognized as a sign of poor management – then motivation dies too.
- Young graduates are differently motivated from their older colleagues; they can also become rapidly demotivated if they're not supported and helped (especially in their first practice), and if they are pushed into positions of unfair responsibility too early.

But motivation – or the lack of it – is not just a problem among the professional staff. Veterinary nurses are highly competent, capable people but their motivation often becomes limited – primarily by their professional career structure. In many cases, the only significant promotional prospects for a veterinary nurse in practice is away from nursing to restricted 'managerial' positions. The promotion is often not accompanied by sufficient recognition of the authority the new position should bring and, coupled with lack of training, results in demotivation and even loss of an excellent staff member from the practice.

Young workers ('twenty-something') have been identified as a motivational challenge (Bradford and Raines, 1992) because their perceptions and expectations are so different from older people. Compared to those in their thirties, forties and fifties, they tend to be self-orientated and cynical, materialistic, and slow to commit themselves to responsibility. They want instant recognition of skills, rapid and easy promotion, and reward in return for their input – *now*. Understanding that these differences exist is the first step for a leader in motivating both his or her young professional and support staff.

## Motivation: accepting responsibility

The purpose of motivation is to stimulate someone to work harder and better: to get performance. This is achieved not through threats and bullying but by encouraging the individual to *accept responsibility* to perform. Drucker (1968) argues that responsibility is the essential internal self-motivation for performance. He also points out that the question of whether people *want* to assume responsibility is irrelevant; an organization *needs* performance which it can only get by encouraging, inducing, and, if need be, by pushing the person into assuming responsibility.

Motivation, then, is getting your staff to accept responsibility for their own performance: successful motivation is getting them to do this willingly and take pride in the results.

To motivate successfully you need to understand what inspires the individual, what makes him or her 'tick'. Do this through finding out what the person wants by asking questions such as:

- What do you like most about your job?
- What do you like least about your job?
- What would you like to do in the future?
- What skills would you like to learn?
- When do you do your best work?
- Who do you enjoy working with the most?
- What is most important about this job for you?

Remember that what motivates you may be very different from what motivates other people. For this reason, 'blanket' motivation such as a practice incentive scheme often does not work well *because* people are motivated by different things.

The three greatest motivators have been identified as money, happiness, and recognition. Money buys things, so it can also provide social recognition and esteem, but money *itself* does not motivate. It motivates only when the person is *ready to assume responsibility*; incentive pay produces better output where there is already a willingness to perform better. Responsibility cannot be 'bought'.

Happiness and what is needed to achieve happiness is complex and best defined by the individual.

Recognition, both socially and from peers, is a very powerful motivator. People will even choose recognition, in the form, say, of a title, over all other motivators.

Having identified the motivating force(s), it is important to recognize and remove the demotivators. In practice, these typically include:

- *Lack of support for actions* – the leader does not support the actions and ideas of an enthusiastic staff member.
- *Lack of confidence* – often arises from past-experience conditioning but can also arise from lack of experience and training.
- *Negative opinions* – the devastating effect of negativity in an organization is discussed in Chapter 5, p. 59.
- *A feeling of 'no future here'* – a situation frequently confronting young, energetic veterinarians who gradually realize the partnership they were promised is not going to materialize.
- *Feeling unimportant* – good management makes everyone feel important.
- *Not knowing what is going on* – good communication systems keep everyone in touch.
- *Being given routine, humdrum work to do* – mixing the mundane with the challenging helps alleviate frustration.
- *Boredom* – a key feature of the successful practice is that people are kept busy (doing constructive things).
- *Overharsh judgement of failure* – everyone makes mistakes. A good manager will help the person learn from the experience in a kindly and supportive way.

The final stage in motivating staff to give desirable performance is by showing them how to get what they want, which must also link with what the practice wants.

# ▪ Performance assessment

*I think it is an immutable law in business that words are words, explanations are explanations, promises are promises – but only performance is reality. Performance alone is the best measure of confidence, competence and courage . . . (As a manager) . . . just remember that:* **Performance is your reality.** *Forget everything else. That is why my definition of a manager is what it is: one who turns in the performance. No alibis to others or to oneself will change that.*
Harold Geneen, ex-Chief Executive, ITT

Performance assessment serves two main functions. It not only is a measure of achievement, but it also helps to develop the individual or team. Performance standards can be set for a variety of different parameters from personality attributes to income generated.

*In a Canadian practice I visited, the two practice principals reviewed their staff's behavioral and attitudinal performance on a monthly basis – and vice versa! A simple questionnaire for each person was completed separately by the staff member and practice principals. The two sets of answers were then compared and adjustments recommended to the person's performance. The questionnaire concentrated mainly on characteristics such as friendliness, politeness, and attitude to colleagues and clients. Each was ranked on a 1–5 scale. Improved performance was rewarded with an end-of-the-month bonus.*

*The practice principals found it very useful as it not only meant they could manage the desirable behaviour of their staff – but also their own.*

To measure performance you need to define the performance you want and agree this with the staff member/team, give suitable training and instruction to enable achievement, agree how and when the performance will be measured and determine what the rewards/penalties are of achievement/non-achievement (see Table 7.2). Clearly, the rewards of performance are the motivators you have already mentioned.

When you decide what the performance is that you seek, you also need to work out a way to measure it. Some performance goals, such as having a pleasant telephone manner, or client satisfaction, can be difficult to measure. Make them as specific as possible; for example, saying please and thank you, and calling the client by name at least twice in a conversation

**Table 7.2** *Setting performance parameters*

- Work with the staff member to identify three or four personal and professional goals that are compatible with the practice mission (see SMART goals, Chapter 2)
- Analyse their ability to achieve these goals
- Define the rewards and penalties for achieving/not achieving the goals
- Agree with the individual how their performance in achieving these goals will be measured
- Give them suitable training and instruction that will enable them to achieve the goals
- Monitor their performance at agreed intervals
- Allow for the learning curve – expect staff members to improve at a pace which matches their own natural aptitude
- Asses their final level of achievement with them and reward or penalize accordingly

might be specifications for the former, while grading different aspects of 'satisfaction', such as speed of telephone answer, cleanliness of practice, friendliness of staff on a 1–5 scale of requirements may be a way of measuring the latter.

Other goals can be easier to measure; for example increase in average transaction fee, number of clients seen, number of dentals performed, or appointment time with clients.

> *It is very important to be very clear about what is to be appraised; for example for a veterinarian required to increase his average transaction fee (ATF) the following should be considered: ATF is the sum of all the fees paid divided by the number of transactions. It can be influenced by the number of services supplied per client, and the amount of prescription and other medical and non-medical goods sold. Which of these do you want the veterinarians to concentrate on? Is the increase in ATF to link with a dental focus, for example? It is important to define exactly what the practice is looking for to avoid mistakes – and frustration on both sides.*

Frequent and regular performance appraisal stops the person drifting away from their performance goals. Either continuous assessment or at least a review every 3 months is recommended. Continual assessment has the advantage that it provides feedback about a situation *at the time it occurs*, not later – and behaviour responds much more quickly to prompt correction or praise than delayed reaction. Three-month reviews are, perhaps, more formal, but may be easier to plan and organize for the inexperienced reviewer.

> *The concept of performance appraisal is new for most veterinarians and there is likely to be some resistance to it initially. It takes time for them to understand what is required, the importance of the regular review – and that it is ultimately very beneficial to their own performance. My advice to principals is to plan carefully: clearly identify the behaviour you want from staff members, and work hard to keep them on track. The results will speak for themselves.*

Concentrate on the task and how well it is performed rather than on personality issues. Give guidance, as and when required, on where and how to improve, and get your staff members to agree on any things they need to do to improve. But don't forget to praise the right behaviour. Prompt praising of the right behaviour is the best way to get more of it.

## ■■■ Incentive schemes

Incentives are rewards that stimulate greater productivity in a specific area. They can reward the individual or the team. They are frequently misused, usually because they are set up so that practice members compete against each other – which disrupts the team and can upset the whole practice.

However, incentive programmes for individuals can be made successful by adhering to the following five rules (Denny, 1993):

- *Everyone must have an evenly weighted chance to win.* There are two important reasons for this:
  If there is little or no chance of winning people will not even try. If a low performing person wins through luck it can be enormously demotivating for a high performing person (e.g. in a raffle draw).
- *Time the incentive system carefully* – short, intense competitions lasting a maximum of 3 months have a more powerful immediate effect than long, drawn out contests.
- *Decide exactly what the scheme should achieve* – then reward the behaviour you seek.
- *Give tangible prizes* – money is not the best incentive in competitions because it so easily 'dissolves' on mundane household and personal items. A tangible prize such as theatre tickets, wine, a

food hamper, and so on are far more effective – and make the tickets or weekends away for two people.

■ *Ensure the scheme is fully understood* – everyone should be able to answer the following questions:

Exactly what do I have to do?
Exactly what do I get?
By when?

To convert this to an incentive programme for a team get members to work towards joint goals that depend on the team working and co-operating together, for example increasing the number of dentals performed in the next month, or increasing the sale of diets by 10% over the course of the year. And reward them jointly.

## ■■■ Delegation

*What percentage of your professional worktime is spent doing things that a more junior person could do, if we got organized and trained the junior to handle it with quality?*
David Maister, Management Consultant

Delegation is a skill veterinarians are notoriously bad at using and yet it is the key to effective management. Delegation means handing the responsibility for a project or situation to a suitably qualified person, to achieve a good outcome. It serves two purposes:

■ It helps relieve your own work load – much of which may be neither necessary nor appropriate that you do anyway.
■ It encourages people to practise self-management and to take responsibility for their own areas/projects.

Delegation can only really be used on people who are sufficiently trained and confident to require minimum support and direction. It is not appropriate for a raw recruit or an inexperienced person. There are two primary levels at which delegation usually occurs in veterinary practice:

■ From principal to veterinary assistant or practice manager.
■ From veterinarian to veterinary nurse.

The first level releases the multi-faceted practice principal for more productive time use (Chapter 3, pp. 35–37). The issues that are delegated could include researching and establishing new preventive health care programmes, developing a specialist field, working out staff schedules, administration, marketing programmes, and so on.

The second level serves to release the veterinary assistant from more mundane procedures, at the same time building up the skills of the nurse (see Table 7.3). Many procedures can be performed more profitably by a support staff member than a veterinarian who has a considerably higher chargeable hourly rate.

### The myths of delegation

Veterinarians are often afraid to delegate because they believe myths such as:

- *'I'll delegate myself out of a job!'* – wrong; the veterinarian now has more time to carry out procedures more suited to his or her skills and training.
- *'It's easier/quicker if I do it myself'* – right; in the short term. But in the long term procedures that can be delegated to, say, support staff are those that are not profitable or particularly satisfying for a veterinarian to perform. They include bandaging, stitch removal, anal gland expression, ear cleaning, general health advice, and so on.
- *'At least I know it's been done right'* – wrong; it will also be done properly if the person is trained well.
- *'There is nothing in it for me'* – right; at the moment. There often is no true incentive to delegate, so the feeling is, why waste the time and effort? *'An incentive scheme for the veterinarians in the practice to encourage and support good veterinary nurse coaching may help solve the problem of reluctancy to invest the coaching and supervision time necessary to achieve successful delegation'* (Jevring, 1994). Establishing a measurable monitoring and reward

**Table 7.3** *Reasons for increasing support staff involvement*

---

- Better service to pet and clients
- Improved practice efficiency
- Enhanced practice income
- More productive use of staff training and experience
- Clients often talk more readily to support staff than veterinarians
- Freeing the veterinarians to carry out more procedures better suited to their level of training
- Increased job satisfaction for staff
- Developing responsibility and commitment of staff to practice standards
- Developing staff skills, e.g. in client relations, marketing, minor surgery, etc.
- Encouraging specialization by support staff

---

system for veterinarians within the practice for their ability to coach junior colleagues and veterinary nurses and achieve performance can encourage them to delegate routine procedures.

## Traditional staffing structure

The typical staffing structure of a veterinary practice is shown in Fig. 7.1. There are a small number of partners or owners, a moderate number of professionals (veterinary surgeons), and a relatively large number of support staff. In Britain, the average practice has four veterinarians (of which one or two are principals), and 10 support staff. Does this traditional type of ratio reduce opportunities for delegation?

Leverage is the term to describe the ratio of junior, middle-level and senior staff in a professional firm's organization or the ratio of support staff to veterinary assistants and principals in veterinary practice. Leverage in a practice varies depending on the stage of the practice life-cycle (see Chapter 2 pp. 17–23; illustrated in Fig. 7.2).

By identifying the ideal staffing structure, practices could select and use staff more efficiently. Thus, an 'expert' practice would need a greater proportion of skilled veterinarians than the 'efficiency' practice, who would function best with a high proportion of veterinary nurses (see Table 7.3).

### When to delegate?

You should delegate when:

- You cannot find sufficient time for your priority tasks.
- You want to develop other practice members.
- The job can be done adequately by other practice members.
- You have more work than you can effectively carry out yourself.

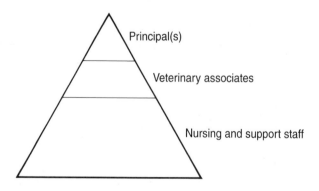

**Fig. 7.1** *The veterinary practice pyramid.*

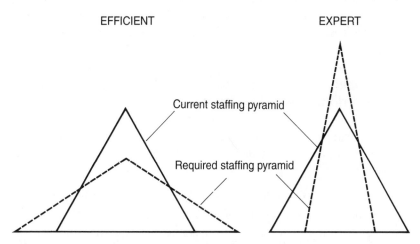

**Fig. 7.2** *The changing staffing requirements of the efficient and expert practice types.*

## How to delegate

> *The only way to develop responsibility in people is to give them responsibility.*
> Blanchard *et al.*, *The One Minute Manager Meets the Monkey*, 1990

Delegation is a learnt skill. There are basically two approaches:

- Tell the person exactly what you want him or her to do, how to do it and what results you expect, so that they are left with little or no room for personal intervention.
- Give responsibility for the results to the person. Focus on results, not methods, and rely on the person's commitment and responsibility to get the job done.

The first method is, in essence, an order. People rarely accept orders out of the Services. The second method takes longer initially, but produces better results and thereby makes you as the manager more effective. Covey (1989) describes five steps to effective delegation:

- *Desired results.* Create a clear mutual understanding of what needs to be accomplished focusing on the *results* not the *methods*; that is, *what* not *how*. Spend time, be patient and clearly visualize the results with the person.

- *Guidelines.* Give minimal guidelines, such as the parameters within which the individual should work, and any known failure paths of the job, so that you are pointing out what *not* to do but not *what* to do.
- *Resources.* Identify and make available all the necessary resources.
- *Accountability.* Define the standards that will be used in evaluating the performance, and fix dates for the evaluation(s) to occur.
- *Consequences.* State clearly what the consequences are, both good and bad, of the evaluation. This could include new job assignments, financial rewards and so on depending on the nature of the job.

Some people are very difficult to delegate to, however patient and persistent you are with them. By refusing to accept responsibility they are refusing to accept the need to produce the performance the practice requires – and their suitability within the practice should be questioned.

## Empowerment

Empowerment is an integral part of delegation. It has been described as *letting go* so that others *get going*; giving people the authority and resources to make better decisions and solve more problems.

> *Consider the common scenario of a receptionist coping with an appointment system that is half an hour behind schedule. If they are empowered to help clients, they will keep them informed about the delay, give the client the option to rebook their appointment or leave their pet for collection later, and will try to make their wait as pleasant as possible by, perhaps, offering coffee or tea and biscuits; or giving them a pair of free film tickets; or giving them a discount on a pet health care product, etc. They are trusted by the practice principal(s) to do all in their power to make this awkward and less than ideal situation pleasant for the client.*

Empowering would be inappropriate for a new graduate or employee who is not familiar with the systems and protocols in the practice, because the core ingredient of empowering is trust; you have to *trust* your staff member's capabilities to be able to empower them. But your belief in their abilities can be reinforced by ensuring they are adequately trained to *be* empowered.

## Summary

1   Performance assessment is critical for increasing the effectivity of both the individual and the team in today's veterinary practice.

2   Motivation, delegation, empowerment, and performance monitoring are key techniques for the practice leader/manager to improve staff performance.

# 8 Achieving Excellence in Client Service

*Quality will be judged by its user, not announced by its maker.*

Lockheed Industries

THE importance of client service, that is serving the needs of clients, is appreciated by most professionals and most professional firms. Banks, legal firms, publishing houses, fast-food firms, travel agencies, hairdressers, hospitals, dental practices, and so on are examples of businesses that exist only to perform services to their customers or clients. Veterinary practice is also a professional service firm, but does your practice provide such excellent service that your clients will never look elsewhere?

Clients cannot judge the level of medical and surgical care you give, but they can and do judge the level of service they receive. As this may be, in the client's eyes, the only major factor that distinguishes you and makes you unique from other practices, striving for excellence in client service is essential.

Client recommendations are very powerful; satisfied clients will recommend you to four or five other people, whereas dissatisfied clients tell nine to ten people. Studies have shown that for every dissatisfied client that does complain, 20 say nothing – they just don't return. Measuring client satisfaction in your practice can help prevent these losses, and maintain a more stable, statisfied client base. (The special characteristics of veterinary services are discussed in Chapter 11.)

## ▬ What is client service?

Client service is the ability to meet client requirements. Services are *experienced*, and the veterinarian's duty, as the service provider, is as much in managing the client's *experience* as in providing technical expertise.

Maister's 'First Law of Service' (1984) summarizes this concept:

Satisfaction = Perception – Expectation

If the client perceives better than expected service then satisfaction is high; but if the service received did not meet expectations then satisfaction is low (see Fig. 8.1).

The aim of the members of a veterinary practice is that *every* client who visits the practice comes away very satisfied with the service they have received. That is the way business is built.

## ◼ What is *quality* client service?

Satisfaction can be extended to include a perception of quality. The highly satisfied client will feel they have received a high quality service, whereas the dissatisfied client will be disappointed by the quality of service.

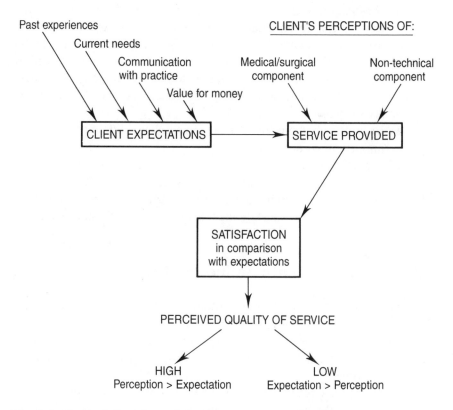

**Fig. 8.1** *Factors influencing satisfaction as a measure of quality.*

## ■■■ Understanding quality

*Quality is more a journey than a destination.*
Anon

Quality is:

- *Made of symbols* such as the friendly smile, the spotless white coat, the pet sent home washed and dried after surgery.
- *Situational* so that different situations require different standards of quality. However, 'high' or 'low' quality does not exist – either the service meets the client's requirements or it does not. Compare a French restaurant with a McDonald's; the French restaurant does not have 'higher' quality than McDonald's because their customers have different needs. Diners in the French restaurant want gourmet food and elegant service; McDonald's customers want good food, cheaply, in a hurry.
- *Dynamic* and constantly requiring reassessment and change. Quality can become dated as requirements change; compare the needs of customers shopping for their weekly groceries in the village high street 40 years ago, where personal service and time to gossip was important, to the customer rushing to the modern supermarket now, where range of goods and speed of checkout are valued.
- *Relative;* what one person perceives as quality may not be as important to another.
- *Attention to detail;* a quality practice must show that quality everywhere at all times. It is not adequate to simply have longer appointments and charge higher fees – the practice must always be spotlessly clean, the staff must always be friendly, and so on.

## ■■■ How do clients define quality?

The measurement of satisfaction/quality is still in a primitive state because there is no standard formula that precisely matches all individual client requirements. In addition, quality is affected by many variables, from individual veterinarian's interpretation of the service to client compliance with instructions.

Research in the USA has produced a new and widely accepted set of 10 client quality evaluation criteria. Although they are for non-professional services, they still help to highlight the importance of identifying quality criteria issues which are *actually* important to clients and that clients really *do* use which are often different from the criteria professionals such as veterinarians *think* are important to clients, and which *they* use to evaluate quality.

- *Reliability* which involves being consistent, dependable and keeping promises.
- *Responsiveness* meaning how quickly and willingly the service is provided.
- *Competence* shown by the contact staff.
- *Accessibility* in terms of both physical accessibility to the service provider, and the friendliness and ease of contact on a personal confrontation basis.
- *Courtesy* including the consideration, politeness and friendliness of the contact staff.
- *Communication* both through making contact with clients and taking time to explain things to them; and through being a good listener to their particular problems.
- *Credibility* which involves honesty, integrity, trustworthiness and reputation.
- *Security* meaning freedom from risk, doubt and even danger.
- *Knowing/understanding the client*: the level of effort made to fully satisfy the individual's needs.
- *Tangibles*: quality is also reflected in tangible elements such as the physical facilities and equipment, personal appearance and attitude of contact staff, and level of fee set.

## Quality control in practice: service cycles

Service cycles are a practical way to apply quality control in your practice (see Figs 8.2–8.4). The method is simple: identify a service and write, in step-wise fashion, what should happen ideally. This is the inner ring of the cycle. Then, for every step, identify all the things that could go wrong. This is the outer ring. By identifying all potential problems you are in a position to control and prevent them before they happen. You are, thus, controlling the quality of service that you give.

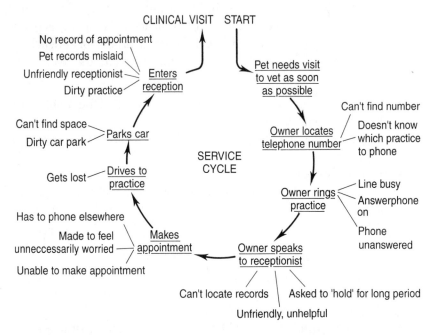

**Fig. 8.2** *The service cycle for a client trying to make a same-day appointment. The main circle represents the 'ideal'; the outer comments are the things that could go wrong.*

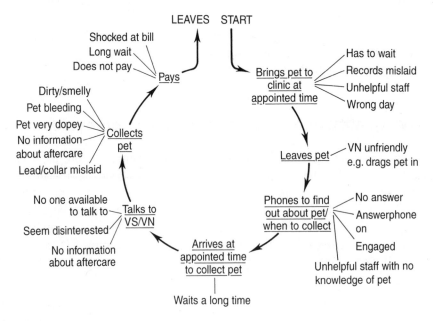

**Fig. 8.3** *The service cycle for a client leaving a pet for elective surgery.*

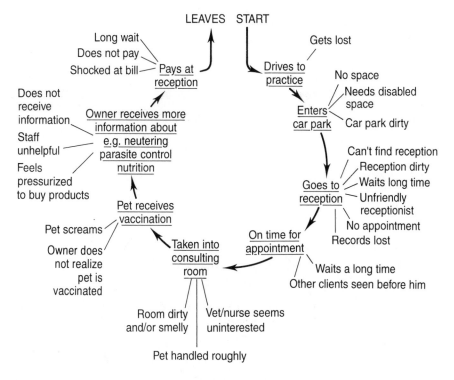

**Fig. 8.4** *The service cycle for a client bringing a pet for vaccination.*

## ■■■■ **How quality of service influences consumers**

When consumers purchase goods three main deciding factors are involved:

- price;
- product quality;
- service quality.

Where the products appear the same, price is the deciding factor. If price is broadly similar then product quality becomes the deciding factor, and if price and product quality are pretty much the same then the quality of service associated with the product is used to select it (see Table 8.1 and Fig. 8.5).

The *generic product* is what the client needs: they need milk, or a new car, or a notebook.

The *enhanced product* is the benefits the product will bring: skimmed milk may taste better than whole milk; a four-door saloon car may be more

**Table 8.1** *Improving the product*

| Product | Generic | Enhanced | Integrated |
|---|---|---|---|
| Milk | Price | Taste | Delivery<br>Packaging<br>Friend's recommendations |
| Pet food | Price | Dog? cat?<br>Palatability | Pet health management<br>Professional recommendation<br>TV advertising |

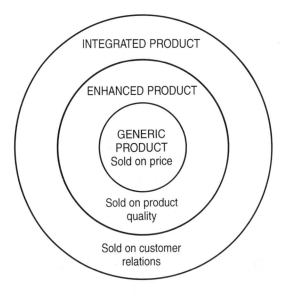

**Fig. 8.5** *What sells a product.*

convenient than a two-door; a hard-backed notebook is more durable than a soft-backed one.

The *integrated product* is everything related to what is being sold. It includes service, word of mouth references, convenience of locality for purchase, the market image of the product, and so on.

Around 20% of people make their buying decision based on price only. The remaining 80% consider the value and benefits of the purchase as well as the price. In today's competitive market service quality is becoming more and more the deciding factor in purchasing goods. It is also becoming very significant in the purchase of services. There is no end-point with the search for quality service – it is a goal that can always be improved upon.

# ■■■■ Client assessment of service

Assessment of the level of service involves a number of factors of variable importance to the client:

- *Practice personnel.* Clients often buy 'people' rather than the service. In hiring the right people to work in veterinary practice you need to ensure they are people-orientated, friendly personalities, and good communicators with experience in dealing with people and their problems. They also need appropriate training for them to do their job well.
- *Quality level.* Quality measurement is important and necessary (see Quality control in practice: service cycles, above).
- *Fee level.* Consumers equate quality with a premium price, for example, Rolls Royce, Rolex watches, and designer clothing, so fees are an important method for clients to judge quality of services high in credence (i.e. those which are difficult for them to evaluate directly). This assessment is based not so much on what they actually pay as what *value* they perceive from the payment. High fees reflect a high self-image in the practice, and are often accepted from professionals with a strong positive image or reputation. Many people prefer higher fees – equating it to better service – where a high risk is perceived.
- *Waiting time.* Clients do not appreciate being kept waiting – their time is valuable to them. Where a wait is necessary, for example if the veterinarian is unavoidably held up with an emergency, informing the client what is happening and giving them the option of waiting or rebooking shows that the practice understands their time is valuable too.
- *Medical and surgical facilities.* The medical and surgical facilities in the practice are part of the service to clients. Of course, if clients are not informed about them (see Chapter 11) they cannot appreciate them. A practice laboratory, for example, is often not cheaper to run than sending samples to a commercial laboratory, but has the major advantage of providing a rapid interpretation service to clients.
- *'Packaging and labelling'.* The way the practice markets itself and communicates its services to its clients is part of the differentiation process that helps clients choose between practices.

## ■ Circles of service

Client service can also be expressed in terms of the generic, enhanced and augmented product. These are circles of service (see Fig. 8.6). The innermost circle represents the generic or core expectations or needs of the client, the next circle is the enhanced or perceptible level of service, and the outer circle represents the augmented or excellent client service. It is this outer level that differentiates practices.

For most people, coming to the 'vet's' is a necessity, not a pleasure. The purpose of striving for the outer or augmented level of service is to make the visit a highly satisfactory experience; the client's perceptions of the service received should be greater than their expectations.

### *Core level: What is the client really seeking for their pet? (see Chapter 2, p. 25)*

In coming to a veterinary practice clients seek:

- Freedom from worry about their pet's health.
- Reassurance that they are doing the right thing for their pet.
- To have access to experts in animal health care.

Every practice provides this generic core.

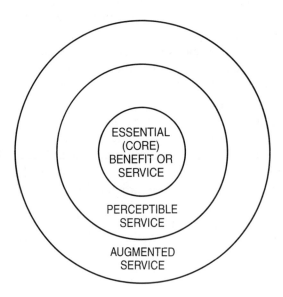

**Fig. 8.6** *Circles of service.*

### Perceptible level of service

This is the standard of client service offered by the majority of practices.

### Augmented service

An increasing number of veterinary practices compete at the augmented service level. It is an opportunity for practice members to really use their imagination to create exceptional service for clients.

Practices functioning at the augmented level are taking veterinary practice out of the basic commodity level and moving it towards a specialized or branded level. In product terms, it is like comparing generic-label products with brand-name products. Some people will seek the generic-label product, others will seek the brand-name product because of its association with quality and value. The more the practice can differentiate itself through quality of service, the more control it has over its own development and progress (see Table 8.2).

## Striving for augmented service

How can you make a client's visit to your practice memorably pleasant? Even if *you* feel your service is better or more sophisticated than your rival practices, if clients *don't see* the difference, they will go back to their basic criteria of evaluation and compare you on a fee basis – and the cheapest fees usually win.

### Barriers to excellence

There are six major difficulties many practices face when trying to provide the best service to their clients:

**Table 8.2** *Improving the service in veterinary practice*

| Service | Generic | Enhanced | Augmented |
|---|---|---|---|
| Vaccination | Price | Health protection | Total health care<br>Peace of mind |
| Euthanasia | Price | Body disposal choices | Care and compassion from staff<br>Euthanasia at home? practice?<br>Client recommendations |

- *Disagreement amongst the practice principals* about the importance and value of quality client service.
- *General undervaluing of the client.*
- *Failure to listen to clients.* Too many veterinarians believe they know what their clients want when only the *client* knows what they *really* want.
- *Indifferent, unmotivated employees.* Where there is little training, empowerment or motivation for delivering service quality excellence staff do not see the value of the extra effort involved. If staff feel they are not valued they see little reason to value the client.
- *Frontline contact staff are powerless to solve most client's problems.* Most clients will stay with the practice if their problem can be resolved immediately. By training and empowering frontline staff to deal with problems – and potential problems – client satisfaction will be much greater.
- *Practice dishonesty.* There are many practices which claim to give good client service but really don't. Quality client service requires vigorous attention to detail. If the practice sets itself up to be the best practice in town it has to be the best practice in town – at everything. It has to be the cleanest, smartest, and most efficient practice, have the best staff, the best facilities, and so on. Clients soon notice if the fees charged are not, in their view, compatible with the service they receive – and they will go elsewhere.

*For example, I visited a companion animal practice that claimed to offer the best service in town – it certainly charged the highest fees. On entering the practice I noticed it was grubby – the floors and walls had not been properly cleaned, and there was fur and dirt around the edges of the floor. The commercial displays were dusty and poorly stocked – and dogs had urinated on the lowest level. In the consulting room the wallpaint was worn and peeling in places; the rubber mat on the consulting table was badly scratched and damaged, and, again, the floors and walls were dirty. Leaflet displays were half-stocked. The vet's writing table was piled high with a jumble of papers, an old coffee cup and a half-eaten sandwich. This practice did not say 'quality' to me and I'm sure it did not to clients either – and they were voting with their feet.*

# ▪️ Planning for excellence in client service

The aims when planning for excellence in client service are:

- To position yourself in a high-quality market niche.
- To develop a high-quality reputation within that niche.
- To constantly manage your image.
- To concentrate your resources across a narrow front –that is, stick with the business you know best and don't try to diversify too much.
- To commit the practice to achieving better outcomes – make your clients so pleased with the caring service they receive that they want to come back.

The first three points all deal with the practice image: how *clients* perceive the practice. It is not enough to simply state that you have a high quality practice – clients have to see that too. Managing the practice image means *constant* attention to detail and *constant* sensitivity to client needs. Lack of commitment to constancy makes today's top practices tomorrow's mediocre ones.

By concentrating on the business you know best and not trying to diversify too much you have more control over what the practice achieves. Clients who are highly satisfied with the outcome of their visit will be very willing to come back to you again.

# ▪️ Valuing the client

> *Clients don't care how much you know until they know how much you care.*

Client service can only begin when the practice accepts that it is a *client-driven* business; that clients, and their pets, are essential to its survival. Veterinarians, however, are often more interested in developing the intellectual and technical aspects of their craft than in being responsive to clients. All too often clients are regarded as rather annoying – and ignorant – interruptions to the day.

Table 8.3 summarizes a 10-point code of attitude to clients. It highlights the importance of the client in the practice – that without clients (and their animals) there is no practice.

**Table 8.3** *Code of attitude to clients*

- Our clients are the most important people in this practice
- We depend on our clients, they do not necessarily depend on us
- Our clients are not an interruption of our work, but the purpose of it
- Our clients do us a favour by contacting us
- Our clients are part of our practice
- Our clients are not simply cold statistics, but flesh and blood human beings with feelings and emotions like our own
- Our clients are not for us to argue or match wits with
- Our clients bring us specific needs – it is our job to satisfy them
- Our clients deserve the most courteous and attentive treatment we can give
- Our clients are the lifeblood of this practice

Adapted from, *Receptionists Rule Ok*, 1992

# The plan of action

The aims cannot be achieved without a detailed plan of action. This plan can be broken down into 10 steps:

- Commitment by practice leaders/principals/managers.
- Internal evaluation of the practice strengths and weaknesses in association with client service.
- Identifying client needs.
- Setting goals and performance measures.
- Putting the client's needs first.
- Staff motivation.
- Empowerment and training.
- Assessing feedback.
- Recognition and rewards.
- Constant monitoring.

## *Commitment by practice leaders/principals/managers*

Focusing on clients is not simply a case of declaring a new policy. It involves change and commitment in the practice's *whole attitude* starting with that of the practice leaders. They are responsible for setting standards, modelling behaviour, committing resources, and communicating their full support and commitment to everyone. And they always have to stay involved.

It is essential to 'walk what you talk'; to lead by example. Telling your staff that you are committed to your clients whereas in reality you ignore them and are rude about them behind their backs gives a dishonest message, and will encourage your staff to behave in the same way. On the other hand, answering the phone yourself, helping an older client to the car, or wiping down a dirty wall when your staff are busy, and praising your staff when you see them doing a good job, encourages your staff to follow your example of commitment to service.

## Internal evaluation of practice strengths and weaknesses

By identifying what you are (or are not) doing currently for your clients you know where you are starting from in improving your service to clients. To do things right means:

- Defining your clients' requirements.
- Turning those requirements into specifications.
- Identifying key indicators that you can track to learn which requirements are met and which are not. For example, a key requirement for clients might be a maximum 5 minutes waiting time. Does your current system achieve this? If not, how can you modify it to reduce waiting time to an acceptable level?

## Identifying client needs

Reality to your clients is the way *they* see things. To get a clear picture of this, ask them:

- Why they come to you for their pet care?
- What do they value about the services and products in your practice?
- What they like and dislike about the practice?
- How you compare to your competitors?
- What you do that annoys, angers, or pleases them?

(See Appendix 3 for research techniques for client feedback.)

Studies in the United States have shown that today's veterinary clients want:

- Full service care for their pets.
- Quality service.
- Easy access to the veterinarian (which may mean offering more flexible hours in the clinic).
- Behaviour services (behaviour problems are the primary cause of euthanasia in young animals).

- Diagnostic services.
- Dental services (including preventive care advice).

How many of these are you providing in your practice? What are *your* clients' needs?

## Setting goals and performance measures

Having done an internal assessment of the current status of the practice, and an external assessment of the clients' needs, the results must be integrated to develop the goals and performar ce measures for client service in the practice. (See Chapter 2, p. 27 for how to define and set goals.) Goals should be clear, simple and easy to measure; they should also be prominently placed in the practice for all to see including, where appropriate, your clients. For example, if you are working to improve your telephone service *tell* your clients. If you introduce a new service such as better laboratory facilities, *tell* your clients. Help them see and understand you are constantly striving to improve your overall service to them show them that they matter to you.

Do not try to do too much at once as it can be confusing and overwhelming. Bigger goals, for example, can be broken into smaller, simpler stages. However, do not strive for less than 100% quality service; 90% quality is not acceptable. Consider a midwife who works at 90% quality performance ('She only drops one in ten babies!'), or a chaffeur driving at 80% quality performance ('He only hit one in five cars today!') – no more acceptable than your practice striving for less than 100% quality.

## Putting the clients' needs first

The change from a work-driven culture to a client-driven culture is very big. It means putting the needs of the client (and their pet) first. Identify client needs by asking them what they'd like – then acting on it.

## Staff motivation

Client relations mirror employee relations. It is important that staff consistently give the caring image you would like them to. The way you treat your staff is the way they will treat your clients. When a client meets a practice member, that member *is* the practice for the client. Sharing practice information with staff, such as monthly income, food sales targets, and progress towards goals helps keep them involved and interested. By making them feel an important part of the practice they will be more motivated to help clients (see Chapter 7, pp. 86–90, Staff motivation).

### Empowerment and training

Staff need training and empowering to do the best for clients. This means they should have the right to make their own decisions to help clients. For example, although it may be a practice policy to have a strict cash-only payment system for clients, the staff member should have the power to waive this for old, established clients who may have forgotten their wallet. (See also Chapter 7, p. 98, Empowerment).

### Assessing client feedback

Face-to-face interviews, random phone calls and mailed questionnaires are three easy methods to ascertain your current level of client service right from the horse's mouth – the clients themselves.

Negative comments and criticisms provide specific opportunities for you to improve your service – they are nothing to fear. They may include things like the pet being returned smelly after a day in hospital, being kept waiting a long time for an appointment, difficulty contacting the practice by phone, difficult access for disabled people – and often clients are too polite to say them directly to you. Many of these problems can be resolved quickly. But what about complaints about 'staff attitude', 'tone of voice on the telephone', being 'unhelpful', and so on? These grey areas can be more difficult to measure and correct – but it is possible and it is *very* important.

The process of assessing client satisfaction should be repeated regularly. By keeping constantly in touch with the clients' level of satisfaction you can nip problems in the bud and give prompt feedback to your staff.

### Recognition and rewards

Part of effective motivation is rewarding and recognizing when people have done a good job or come up with an innovative and exciting idea. Reward can be anything from a simple 'Thank you' to a cash bonus, but it should be open to everyone. Encouraging staff members to congratulate each other also helps a team work together.

### Constant monitoring

It is not enough to set up a service improvement system and then leave it.

It needs constant reassessment and monitoring to remain truly effective and ahead of the competition. Go back to the circles of service – you are aiming for the outer edge.

# ■■■■ And quality of health care?

> *Health care is not a product or a simple service that can be standardized, packaged, marketed, or adequately judged by consumers according to quality and price.*
> A. Relman, Professor of Medicine and of Social Medicine, Harvard Medical School

Although quality and quality service have been dealt with fairly extensively in this chapter, it is important not to lose sight of the fact that a veterinarian's prime role is, and always will be, in treating animals. Veterinary medical care is a highly personal and individualized service, the true value and success of which can be fully appreciated only by individuals in their individual circumstances.

> *Business managers don't understand why they shouldn't be able to get reliable information about quality of care, which they can weigh against the prices charged. The fact is that the measurement of quality is in a primitive state and is likely to remain so for the forseeable future. Here is the best definition of high quality medical care that I can come up with: it is the care given to a particular patient under particular circumstances by a compassionate and competent physician who has access to consultants and the best current information, who is not influenced by economic incentives to do more or less than is medically appropriate, and who is committed to serve the patient's best interests guided by the latter's wishes and medical needs. This definition emphasizes the physician's key role in allocating medical resources and preserving standards of quality.*
> Relman, *ibid*

This is equally applicable to the practice of veterinary medicine. It is difficult to quantify but it should never be devalued by greed or selling unnecessary services.

## ■ Conclusion

Achieving excellence in client service is like people's desire to stop smoking, or to lose weight. They know and want the goal, they know how to do it, and they know it's worth doing – *but* they don't like putting up with the temporary discomfort to achieve a long-term goal. Client service is not a 'frill', nor is it merely problem-solving, so education and training of staff alone is not adequate. Helping people achieve the aim of excellence in client service means helping them find the self-discipline they need – which means a well thought-out programme or system is necessary. Developing a monitoring system in your practice may create short-term discomfort, and will certainly require disciplined changes in daily life-style, but it will encourage practice members to live up to the goals to which they have agreed, and give excellent client service.

## ■ Summary

1  Veterinary practice is a professional service business.

2  Client service is satisfying client needs.

3  Client service is the major distinguishing factor between practices for clients.

4  Client satisfaction = perception – expectation

5  Quality is an integral part of excellent client service but is not always easy to measure.

6  Excellence in client service can be planned for.

# 9 Preventive Health Care Programmes in Veterinary Practice

*Today's veterinarian measures professional success not by the number of 'interesting' diseases or syndromes diagnosed and treated, but by the number of animals in the practice that are enjoying perfect health because of diligent risk factor management by the caring team of owner and veterinarian.*

Elisabeth Hodgkins, Veterinary Nutrition Consultant

PREVENTIVE health care (PHC) programmes have been well established in farm animal practice for many years. Recognizing that disease prevention is more economically sound for the farmer than disease treatment, herd and flock health schemes have proved an effective way to maintain animal health. Preventive medicine forms the medical and financial backbone of thriving farm animal practice.

These days, the family pet is the family friend. Owners want their pet to have a long and healthy life – they want to prevent illness in their pets. Clients are better informed about their own health and they seek quality health care for their pets too.

Companion animal practice, however, lags behind in preventive health care, partly because the veterinary profession itself has continued to foster the idea that the veterinary surgery is the place to bring sick animals rather than healthy ones. Constantly improving and exciting new medical and surgical techniques mean that emphasis has been put on disease treatment – disease prevention has been largely ignored or forgotten. Now, better medical knowledge about the origins and management of many common diseases makes PHC more applicable than ever before.

# ■■■■ What are preventive health care programmes?

PHC programmes are a co-ordinated attempt to manage and prevent disease. They include the concept of 'risk factor management', defined as examining 'those factors of sickness which can be managed or permanently removed from the still healthy individual, thereby reducing the likelihood that costly diagnostics or treatment will be needed' (Hodgkins, 1990).

PHC programmes run alongside the everyday emergencies and problems of normal practice. They interlink with each other so that, for example, an elderly cat that comes in for its annual booster vaccination can be recommended to join the senior programme, and from there be directed into the dental health care programme.

Programmes have in common a strong component of owner education through regular, frequent contact with clients. This not only strengthens the bond with the client and improves the animal's health, it also enhances practice income. Preventive health care is better quality medicine and quality medicine is profitable.

# ■■■■ Some ground rules

There are four essential ground rules to setting up effective PHC programmes in practice.

### ▨▨▨ *Everyone in the practice must agree on the ethos behind the programmes and be committed to it*

For many practitioners the change over to PHC is difficult. It lacks the glamour of, say, pioneer surgery. However, it is negligent not to practice preventive health care at every opportunity. Giving the animal the chance to be wholly well through good nutrition, and a healthy lifestyle, helped by regular vaccination, neutering, good diet and regular health examinations is the most important way that we can work as a profession for the animals in our care.

### ▨▨▨ *Client education is a key component (see also Chapter 5, Veterinarians as teachers)*

The aim of PHC programmes is to improve animal health through owner education. Gaining the compliance of animal owners is essential to the success of PHC programmes as it is the animal owner who, largely, creates the environment for the animal. This requires a sensitive approach to the owner rather than a dogmatic, 'I am right, you are wrong' attitude.

> *For example, obesity, is the most common nutritional disorder of pets. It results from the animal eating too many calories for its needs. Management is easy – if the veterinarian can gain the full understanding and co-operation of the pet owner. Owners often cannot 'see' that their pet is fat; they believe, 'Fat is happy'; they associate the giving of food with the receiving of love from their pet; they may have obesity problems themselve , and so on. These complex psychological factors combine to make this a tricky and sensitive issue for the veterinarian to deal with successfully.*

The veterinarian must adopt the role of 'teacher' rather than 'fixer'. Client education is a long-term goal – changing client attitudes is not something that happens overnight.

### Good planning is essential to success

Where programmes fail it is always due to unrealistic expectations, lack of organization, and not having clear aims for the programme. Planning (what are our aims? who will be involved? when will we run it? how do we measure success? etc.) takes time initially but ensures a far more successful and satisfactory outcome for all concerned.

### Existing programmes should be updated and improved before new programmes are introduced

Building up a step-by-step range of PHC programmes, starting by revising and updating the ones you currently have in the practice (such as puppy/kitten care), means that clients get the best from each programme before new ones are introduced, and that the practice does not become overwhelmed with too many new projects at once.

## Types of 'wellness' programmes

There are many different programmes that can be established in companion animal practice. These include:

- vaccination;
- puppy and dog health;
- kitten and cat health;
- behaviour management;
- neutering;
- obesity management;
- dental disease;
- senior health care.

# Planning a preventive health care programme

The exact details differ from programme to programme (see Table 9.1 and Table 9.2) but the following approach is a logical and useful basic guide.

**Table 9.1** *Aims for specific programmes*

**Paediatric Health Care**
To educate and inform owners about all aspects of home care of their puppy or kitten including the importance of correct nutrition, dental prophylaxis, exercise, grooming, disease and parasite control, neutering and behaviour management.

**Senior Health Care**
To educate and inform the owners of older animals (over the age of 5–7 years) about the control and management of age-related disorders such as organ failure, dental disease, and joint and skeletal problems through correct nutrition, dental care, exercise and screening for early detection of disease.

**Dental Prophylaxis**
To educate and inform owners about the problems associated with dental disease and how they can be prevented through careful home-management. Special attention is given to animals in high risk categories such as toy breeds, and brachycephalic breeds.

**Behaviour Management**
To educate and inform owners about the benefits of owning a well-behaved pet, and to supply expert advice about management of behaviour problems.

**Obesity Management**
To educate and inform owners about the risks associated with obesity and how they can help prevent or manage the condition in their pets through dietary management and exercise.

**Annual Health Checks**
To educate and inform owners about the benefits of regular screening of a range of parameters, coupled with advice about correct nutrition, and other health maintaining factors to maintain an optimal health status for their pets.

**Table 9.2** *Suggestions for special equipment checklist*

**Paediatric Health Care**
  Weighing scales
  Model demonstrating dental disease
  Toothpaste, toothbrushes
  High-quality growth diet
  Preserved parasite specimens
  Diagrams and specimens of external and internal parasites

**Senior Health Care**
  Weighing scales
  Refractometer
  Laboratory facilites for haematology and blood biochemistry
  Radiographic facilities (ECG; endoscope, etc.)
  High-quality diet to meet the special nutritional needs of older pets

**Dental Prophylaxis**
  Dental scaler and polisher and/or appropriate hand instruments
  Toothbrushes and toothpaste
  Recommended dental chews
  Model demonstrating dental disease
  Appropriate high-quality (dry) diets

**Behaviour Management**
  Appropriate aids to behaviour management
  Suitable high-quality diet (diet may be a significant factor in some forms of
  behavioural abnormality)

**Obesity Management**
  Weighing scales
  Weight comparison charts
  Weight-reducing diet
  Weight management diet

**Annual Health Checks**
  Weighing scales
  Refractometer
  Laboratory facilities for haematology and blood biochemistry
  Model of dental disease
  Appropriate high-quality diets
  Diagrams and specimens of external and internal parasites

## Ascertain the need for a programme

Veterinarians are often not sure about introducing PHC programmes into a practice, believing owners will not want them. But it is *not* adequate to rely only on your own feelings about what clients do and do not want. You do not perceive pet health as your clients do. You need to ask your clients what *they* want, and *listen* to their replies. Discussing successful programmes with colleagues in other practices can also be an encouraging pointer.

### Be realistic

PHC is a long-term commitment. Establishing PHC in your practice usually represents a change in attitude not only within the practice, but also in how your clients perceive your practice. It is therefore natural that not all your clients will be immediately interested. PHC programmes not uncommonly fail in practice because of unrealistic and overoptimistic expectations about how many clients will take up the programmes, and how immediate that response will be. For example, with a senior programme, although around 40% of your clients' pets may fall into the senior category, probably well under 10% will initially take up a senior health care programme. On the other hand, with a good recall system you can anticipate an almost 100% response and uptake from your clients on, say, a vaccination programme over the course of the year (see below, the effect of marketing).

### Reasons for starting a programme

Why are you starting a new PHC programme? Has new technical information recently been published which you want to share with your clients? Are you planning to improve the standard of health care offered by the practice? Is this an opportunity to enhance practice income? Do you want to justify the purchase of a new piece of equipment by incorporating its use into a PHC programme? Do you want to utilize staff time more effectively?

### Aims

By assessing your true reasons for wanting to develop a new programme you gain a clearer view of your aims, and how you can measurably achieve them. In general terms your aims will include:

- Improved health of the pets in your care leading to better life quality and greater longevity.
- Better client service through better pet care.
- Improved practice image through practising better veterinary medicine.
- Improved use of staff time and experience.
- Better use of practice facilities.
- Increased income for the practice through increased sales of services.

Work out these aims in terms of SMART objectives (see Chapter 2), that is:

- Specific.
- Measurable.
- Action-orientated.
- Realistic.
- Time-limited.

An example of a specific SMART objective for a dental health programme could be:

> *We aim to examine the mouth of every pet that is presented to the practice and perform dental procedures as necessary on at least 20% of them over the next year. Simultaneously, we aim to give every client in the practice a brochure about dental health care for their pet and will measure the effect of our dental awareness programme by response to a client questionnaire after 6 months.*

### Benefits

> *The promotion of the service needs to be in the form of the BENEFITS of the service rather than the promotion of the service itself. Through promotion, the sale should be made at the programme level rather than at an individual service level, promoting the total health programme rather than a single vaccination or bag of dog food.*
> Dennis McCurnin, Veterinary Management Consultant, 1988

Listing the benefits of the new programme to the practice, the staff, the clients and the pets serves two functions:

- It clarifies why you want this programme and what you hope to get out of it.
- It helps your staff identify the benefits they should discuss with the client – which is how the programme is best promoted.

First and foremost the animals in your care benefit with improved life quality and expectancy. Periodontal disease, for example, affects more than 85% of animals over the age of 3 years (Emily and Penman,1990). It can be effectively managed by a rigorous control programme combining routine clinical examinations and home care, ideally starting from the puppy or kitten's first visit to the surgery.

Around 25% of dogs in the UK are obese (Bush, 1992), and are thus at risk of developing locomotory disorders and joint disease, diabetes mellitus, circulatory problems and certain types of neoplasias. Obesity can be prevented through counselling owners about the seriousness of the disease, and instigating better feeding habits for their pets.

In the United States, behaviour problems are the primary reason for euthanasia of dogs between weaning to maturity. In the UK in 1990, it was noted by members of the Association of Pet Behaviour Counsellors that most of the 3000 cases treated were recognized as having been avoidable had the pet been purchased from a better source and socialized properly with its own kind and people during critical weeks of development prior to about 18 weeks of age. Raising breeder and client awareness of the importance of having a well behaved, well socialized pet through running behaviour advisory programmes can help prevent unneccessary pet deaths.

Pet owners benefit from PHC programmes by having a happier, healthier pet. Through increased awareness of the risks that can lead to disease, they can make more informed decisions about their pet's health and, in the long term, save money on the potentially expensive cost of treatments of preventable conditions.

The practice benefits in many ways from PHC programmes. For example, staff gain more satisfaction from practising better medicine and enjoy the increased responsibility from more personalized client contact – and practice profit can significantly increase through more productive use of trained staff time plus sales of quality health products. These profits can, at least in part, be ploughed back into the practice for further development and improvement of client services.

## *What do we need?*

All programmes require a committed attitude from the whole practice, appropriately trained staff, suitable client education materials (information brochures, personalized letters, demonstration models, practice photograph file, illustrative material, etc.), appropriate pet health record cards (e.g. one where the weight can be marked on a graph for an obesity programme, or where the major problem areas in a mouth can be illustrated for a dental programme), a reminder/recall system and appropriate dietary management.

Without doubt PHC programmes are easier to run if the practice has computerized client records. Not only can clients be easily targeted (dog/cat owners, high risk breeds, senior health checks), but the remainder/recall system is also more easily instigated.

Some programmes may require an investment in certain types of equipment such as a dental scaler and polisher, weighing scales or laboratory equipment (see Table 9.2). As these can be used in many different ways in the practice they represent a worthwhile outlay.

### The cost of caring

The potential profit from setting up and running a new programme can be roughly calculated as follows.

Outgoing expenses:

- Planning time.
- Staff training.
- Staff time to run the programme.
- Employing an expert, for example in pet behaviour.
- Production of promotional literature (newsletters, handouts, reminders, posters, etc.).
- Mailing costs.
- Purchase of special equipment (weighing scales, laboratory equipment, dental instruments).
- Purchase of professional OTC products (diet foods, dental home-care prophylactic products, behaviour management products, etc.).

Income:

- Direct client uptake of services and products.
- Continued, long-term use of specific products such as foods, dental products.
- Indirect effect of uptake of other services and products, such as medical or surgical procedures following the primary service (e.g. vaccination leading to laboratory tests and wart removal).

The profitability to the practice is enhanced by allowing support staff to run these programmes. This not only gives them the opportunity to create their own additional income for the practice but it also releases the veterinary surgeons for procedures more suited to their skills and training. In addition, clients are often more willing to talk freely to staff members and are more likely to ask them about other services available for the better health of their animals.

### Fee-setting

The fee charged for the programme should accurately reflect the time and expertise involved. Fees are often used as a measure of quality, so a high fee often represents high quality to the client. However, setting the fee is a major stumbling block to establishing PHC programmes in many practices. Do not be ruled by your own 'fee comfort factor'. Calculate all the costs involved and express this as a package. Explain the *benefits* of the programme and how it can help the health of the pet to convince interested owners of the value of the fee. Remember that you are appealing to the 80% of people whose buying decision is not ruled only by price, but who consider value and benefits too. (See Appendix 1 for more about fees and fee-setting).

## Marketing

> *The services that veterinarians think their clients don't want, most clients **won't** want. Why? Because they don't **know** the services are available.*
> Don Dooley, Veterinary Management Consultant, 1992

For the new programme to work, clients must know about it. The response to any programme depends partly on how enthusiastically you and your staff market it. For your staff to be keen and committed they require an *understanding* of the programmes' aims, and additional coaching in how to market them to clients. For example, relying solely on a targeted letter to clients will probably give less than a 10% response rate, whereas a letter plus a phonecall from a trained member of staff can boost the response to a much higher level. Some or all of the following methods of promoting a programme to your clients can be considered:

- Train your staff to identify opportunities to TALK to clients about the new service.
- Make a display in the practice using promotional literature and posters.
- Target mail information to clients.
- Use reminders (written and telephone).
- Print articles in the practice newsletter.
- Encourage features on local TV and radio stations – local newspapers may be interested in a brief article promoting the concepts of preventive health.

## The importance of client education (see also Chapter 5, p. 60)

PHC programmes are, essentially, client education programmes, teaching animal owners that many conditions are preventable rather than simply treatable. A common example of the success of owner education is how regular vaccination has reduced the incidence of canine hepatitis, leptospirosis, distemper and parvovirus.

Where specific disease conditions have been pin-pointed it has been relatively easy to focus on their prevention, for example hereditary eye disease, hip dysplasir. But problems such as inappropriate behaviour, and ageing changes are 'grey' topics that are less specific, and more difficult to measure. Ageing, of course, is not preventable and ultimately results in death. However, ageing changes can largely be *managed*, which can give the older animal a better quality and more comfortable life. Topics like these offer special challenges to communicate the benefits of PHC programmes clearly to clients.

## When and where?

When are you going to carry out the procedures in the programme? Can the animals be booked in for quieter times in the day such as late morning and early afternoon, perhaps during the middle of the week? Will the animals need to be admitted? How long will the procedures take? Whose time will be involved? Is there a separate room where the VN can carry out examinations and client discussions? Should you aim to start this programme in a quieter period of the year?

Different programmes take different amounts of time and may need to be performed in different places. For example, pet behaviour counselling needs around 2 hours per consultation, a high degree of owner involvement and often requires a home visit, whereas a senior health programme mainly uses trained support staff time in taking samples, and giving much of the general health care advice. Be careful not to limit yourself by restricting yourself only to the times immediately convenient to the practice – these are often quiet times *because* they are not convenient to owners.

## Developing a protocol

A protocol for the programme is essential. It should be clearly and concisely worked out. Consider the following points:

- How to identify the pet for whom the programme is suitable.
- How to explain the benefits to the owner and gain their commitment.
- How the owner will participate, for example what they do at home such as dietary management, teeth-cleaning, training.
- The role of the veterinary surgeon.
- The role of the support staff.
- The role of external experts.
- Recommending health care products and their use.

Medical and treatment decisions lie with the clinical staff, but support staff will have valuable suggestions on how to make the programme run smoothly and effectively. A trial run of the programme in its entirety using a colleague's pet or a co-operative client can iron out any problems before introducing it into the practice.

## Personnel training

Well-informed and motivated staff – and that includes the veterinarians – are vital to the success of a PHC programme. Motivate staff by involving them in the programmes from the beginning, and empowering them to run them according to goals they have helped define.

Educate staff using both internal and invited external speakers. For example, the representative from a vaccine company can describe the use of the vaccines for a vaccine programme, or a veterinary nutritional expert from a pet nutrition company can explain the importance of dietary management in a senior, obesity or puppy programme. Discuss the best laboratory tests to perform with the university experts; invite a pet behaviour specialist to work with the practice. Recommend relevant scientific papers that staff members should read; talk to colleagues who are running similar programmes.

Discuss the application of the new knowledge in practical terms. How can your staff best use this information? Can you delegate the day-to-day management of the programme to a staff member? How can this information be phrased in client communications? Is it practical (and ethical) to perform every single recommended test? Can you confidently interpret results? How do you handle client objections? How do you identify opportunities to promote the programme? Find out the potential problems and pitfalls and work out how you can overcome them. By finding answers to these questions *before* you even start, your programme has more chance of success.

Finally, reward your staff with praise and a share of the profits.

### Measuring the effect of the programme

There is little point in setting up a new programme if no method is used to measure how effective the programme is, and how practice income is improved. The effect of the new programme can be determined directly from the number of clients that take up the new service, and the increase in related product sales. Indirect measurements include calculating support staff productivity levels and through questionnaires to measure client satisfaction.

## Summary

1   PHC is challenging and profitable.

2   PHC benefits animal health through disease prevention and helps bond clients to the practice.

3   PHC is practising better medicine.

# 10 Professional Retailing in Practice

*Any business that wants to succeed must be aware of its customers' requirements ... failure to do so is a missed opportunity to satisfy client needs and to maximize profits.*

Geoff Little, Senior Practice Partner

SELLING means the promotion of services or products through their benefits so that a consumer is persuaded to buy. It is something we all do all the time on both a personal and professional level. We 'sell' our ideas and beliefs to our friends and by clever argument persuade them of their value. We 'sell' ourselves to our clients by convincing them, through our professionalism, of the benefit of employing us to treat their pet. We 'sell' laboratory tests, courses of antibiotics, and surgical operations through the benefits they will offer the health of the pet. Similarly, we are constantly 'buying' based on appreciation of benefits. We 'buy' our friends' ideas. We choose to buy selected medicinal products, disposable items, and technical equipment for our practices, and have the practice cars serviced at a particular garage because of the perceived benefits to the practice.

Professional retailing – that is, the selling of professional goods – is still, for many veterinarians, a controversial issue. They are not sure how to retail and they associate selling with the old-fashioned image of the pushy salesperson with dubious morals. Retailing is a skill that involves personnel education, stock management, labour costs, advertising, administration, employee time, facility management, insurance, and so on. Veterinarians who learn about retailing products and services profitably find it is a logical step to then retail the products they are verbally recommending rather than refer owners somewhere else.

Veterinarians need to look at pet care from the client's point of view – today's time-pressured clients increasingly seek 'one-stop shopping', and once a sick pet is treated, they want to know when to bath the dog, or how to manage its smelly breath. By not only giving this advice but also selling the appropriate professional health care products under the same roof, the practice is giving 'added value' service to the client – an important component of excellent client service.

## ■■■■ The benefits of retailing

Retailing quality professional products from veterinary practices has many benefits:

- increases practice income;
- increases opportunity for building a good relationship with clients through frequent return visits and increased client contact;
- can largely be done by trained members of staff;
- is better use of trained staff time;
- is part of total health care service;
- provides a welcome service to clients.

Retailing professional goods increases practice income both directly and indirectly. For example:

- Premium quality petfoods for both therapeutic use and feeding healthy animals make a very significant difference to practice income in many practices (from 10 to 30% of income can be generated by sale of these products) as well as improving animal health.
- Through more efficient and productive use of time, trained staff can become profit centres within the practice.
- The increased client contact through repeat sales increases the opportunity for more business with the client.

## ■■■■ The downside of retailing

Many veterinarians are resistant to the concept of retailing in their practices. They feel that it detracts from the professional image of the practice, makes the practice look commercial and money-orientated, and reduces the caring image fostered in the clinic.

These objections are often based on misconceptions such as:

- 'We have to have large display!'.
- 'We haven't got room for a display!'.
- 'I don't want to look like a pet-shop!'.
- 'Selling is unprofessional!'.

- 'It isn't profitable!'.
- 'We don't know what to stock!'.
- 'I'm a vet – I don't want to sell things!'.

My responses to these objections are covered in the remainder of the chapter. A recent American study made a strong case for the retailing of quality petfoods for veterinary practices – 34 average veterinary hospitals in six States investigated the profitability of quality petfood sales in the practices, and found that the profits from food as a percentage of the hospital-wide profits averaged 10.9% which came from 3.3% of the hospital's total area, and took 3.3 hours per week (equivalent to 8.3% of one full-time equivalent support staff member) (unpublished data from Hills Pet Nutrition, Inc.). I am sure that surveys of other professional health care products would reveal similar, highly profitable results.

## ■■■■ Is retailing professional?

Yes. Veterinary professional retailing is helping the client make an informed decision about which health care products are best for their pet. There is nowhere better that clients can get this information than from the animal care experts – the veterinary profession. Many of the products sold in practice form an integral part of preventive health care programmes. Selling quality health care products enhances the bond of trust between the client and the practice – not only is the practice providing reliable, effective products, but the client also returns more often to the practice for further purchases, which allows deeper development of the client–practice bond. The ultimate result is that everyone benefits – the pet is healthier, the client is happy, the practice is more profitable – and it is giving better professional service.

## ■■■■ Is retailing ethical?

Professional retailing is only unethical if it is done unethically – that is, if products are sold that do not benefit the animal or if they sold in a way that is unethical, but selling quality products of benefit to animal health to the correct recipients can only be right.

If you are still not convinced, ask your clients what they want – would they *like* you to supply reliable, high-quality health care products for their animals? Or do they prefer to go to the supermarket or petshop?

# ■ Planning professional retailing

To be successful, retailing in practice needs careful planning. Ask yourself the following questions:

- *Why do we want to retail?* Does it improve our service to our clients? Can we do a better job of caring for animals? Can we increase practice profits?
- *What do we want to retail?* Professional health care products such as premium petfoods, flea products, anthelminitics, behavioural aids, general care products (cat carriers, litter trays, food bowls, nail clippers, etc.)?
- *Who will do the retailing and how?* Do our staff need extra training?
- *How will we measure the success of our retail business?* Increase in practice profits? Increase in average transaction fee?
- *When will we do the retailing and where?* In the reception area? In the consulting room?

Make a plan of action that answers these questions and give yourself a timescale to set up a retail system within which to work. Start with a limited range of top-selling products that you are confident about (your distributor should be able to help you identify these) and build up the system.

# ■ Selling is communication

Successful retailing comes from good communication. Good communication starts with trust – if a client trusts you and the members of your practice they are more likely to accept your recommendations (see Creating trust, Chapter 4, p. 49).

As described in detail in Chapter 4, and in Chapter 11 in relation to marketing services, communication uses all the senses, especially sight, hearing, smell and touch. To make professional retailing in your practice effective, enhance your selling technique by using these senses.

- *Sight* – product displays, posters, handout information/product brochures.
- *Hearing* – talk to clients about the products, use videos to endorse your message.
- *Smell* – allow clients to smell products such as shampoos and deodorants before purchasing them.

■ *Touch* – arrange displays so that clients can handle products before purchase (see below, Making an effective display).

## The art of selling

Professional retailing is about helping clients. It is based on identifying a need in your clients and satisfying it with the product(s) at your disposal. There are many books written about selling, and several commercial veterinary companies have seminars to teach selling techniques so it is not my intention to describe it in detail here, but the basic steps to successful selling are:

■ *Identifying opportunities for sales* – of almost 3 million flea collars sold in the UK in 1990, only 6% were sold through veterinary surgeries. This represents a huge missed opportunity to veterinary practices for client education, better pet care, and improved income.

■ *Identifying client needs through questions and listening to the answers* – by specifying the exact needs the practice can more effectively help the client.

■ *Learning features and benefits of the products for sale* (see below).

■ *Overcoming client objections to convert a negative response to a positive* – most objections arise from a lack of understanding. Use aids such as information brochures and videos to reinforce the message you give verbally, and clarify the benefits of the product to the owner.

■ *To support and comfort the buying decision* – make the client feel they are doing the right thing for their pet when they buy the product(s).

## Features and benefits: the 'So what?' factor

The key to 'selling' is to identify features and benefits. A feature is a characteristic of a product or service; a benefit is how it will help the animal and owner. The two are linked by silently asking the 'So what?' question. By looking at all the products you sell and asking this question you can identify the benefits that you will use to recommend these products to clients. This same technique can also be used to sell services to clients (see Chapter 9, p. 124).

- *We recommend x-brand flea-spray because it not only kills fleas but the eggs as well* (feature).
  *So what?*
  *By regular spraying every three months, you can keep your home and pets flea-free* (benefit).
- *Fido is 10 now and we would recommend he starts on y-brand senior food to slow down ageing changes* (feature).
  *So what?*
  *By giving Fido* y-brand *senior food, you will help him to a longer, healthier life* (benefit).
- *We believe Nogg's nail-clippers are the best available* (feature).
  *So what?*
  *We recommend them to all cat-owners because they are safe and easy to use* (benefits).

## ■■■■ Making staff more effective at selling

Even though it may be the support staff who do most of the selling, it is important that both professional and support staff are involved in professional retailing in the practice. The following are some suggestions for making staff more effective at selling:

- *Sound product knowledge.* Most veterinary product companies are willing to provide training in their products. Product knowledge includes at least a basic knowledge of similar competitor products, the answers to common questions clients may ask, and knowing where to go for further information and references. It goes without saying that if a staff member is unable to answer a client's questions they probably will not sell the product.
- *Knowledge of sales techniques.* These same companies usually teach selling techniques too. A knowledge of the techniques makes staff more effective in communicating the benefits of the products to the client and completing a sale.
- *Major features and benefits of products.* It is the benefits related to the features that sell products, so work together to make a list of three to five features and associated benefits for all the products you sell and make sure all staff are familiar with them to be able to talk to clients. Remember to consider the features and benefits from the clients' point of view – what do they want from a product?
- *Ensure staff use the products on their own pets.* Personal recommendation is extremely powerful. It makes a nonsense of

retailing high-quality pet health care products from the practice if practice members *do not* use them on their own pets.

■ *Encourage a one-to-one staff–client relationship.* By encouraging nurses in the practice to specialize in certain areas, such as dental care, dietary management, puppy/kitten care and so on, the nurse can be used to establish a one-to-one relationship with clients. This personal contact, whom the client knows by name and can ring for further help and information, builds good relations far more quickly than any other system. Because the client comes to know and trust the nurse, they will buy the products. The dental nurse can then, for example, demonstrate how to brush Fido's teeth to his owner, and explain that the toothbrushes and special veterinary toothpaste are available from the clinic. Similarly, when giving worming advice it can be pointed out that effective anthelmintics are available from the practice.

## ▉▉▉ Overcoming common objections

Price often appears to be a client's first concern. The skilled staff member can effectively convert *price* to *value* by talking about benefits. Price becomes a secondary consideration when the client understands/appreciates the benefits of the product to themselves or their pets. Sometimes price needs explaining, for example where a petfood appears expensive per sack but the feeding cost per day is less than or comparable with other brands of food.

Objections are based on lack of understanding. It is important to convey to clients that the products they buy from a veterinary practice really do the job they are supposed to – the client is, then, buying peace of mind.

## ▉▉▉ To whom do you sell and when?

Focus your merchandizing efforts on the 20% of clients that supply 80% of your business. They are not only the least likely to have image problems related to merchandizing in the practice, but they are also the most receptive to your suggestions.

Look for opportunities to recommend products to clients. Vaccination time (worming, flea-control, nutrition), admittance for dental procedures (dental care products, flea control, nutrition), and post-operative care (litter tray and cage for a cat, nutrition, bedding) are all examples of when items can be marketed.

It may not be practical to attempt to discuss, say, nutrition with a harassed mother with a howling babe-in-arms, dog wrapped round her ankles, and a toddler demanding the toilet. However, the old lady with a new kitten and time on her hands is likely to appreciate an explanation of the importance of good nutrition, and worming, and be interested to buy the best products for her pet. Choose your clients but do not discriminate between them – that is, do not assume that they are not interested. Even a simple information leaflet to be read in the peace of their own home can be effective in promoting interest.

Not everyone will buy products, but make it easy for them – make the products and their value as clear as possible using displays and leaflets.

## ■■■■ A few words of warning

The profitability of professional retailing in the practice may be measured in several ways but it is neither professional nor, in the long term, profitable to concentrate purely on profit and more or less force every client to purchase something before they leave the practice. This is *not* good professional retailing.

> *I once spent a long time chatting to an interested client about a particular product I thought would be of benefit to their pet. Their final comment, albeit light-heartedly said, was, 'Allright, I'll buy it. You're a good salesperson!'. I was embarrassed – for the client to feel in anyway pressurized into buying was not my intention.*

The best way for the veterinarian to retail professionally is to use personal recommendations of the product ('I feed this to my dog/ use this on my cat . . .', etc.) coupled with a brief reference to the benefits of using the product for the pet in question. Retailing becomes less and less profitable (and more and more like the dreaded pushy salesman) the longer that it is necessary to spend persuading a client to buy the product.

## ■■■■ Making an effective product display

The aim of a product display is to catch the attention of people and, through projecting a favourable image, influence them to buy. There is a whole 'science' behind what makes an effective display, from the discrete display in the corner of a consulting room through to the massive displays in multi-million-pound turnover supermarkets. All the senses are used in buying.

*For example, to maximize your purchases in a supermarket:*

- *People automatically look left on entering a building, so fresh product displays are sited to the left of the entrance. This also promotes the concept of health, and natural products.*
- *The smell of fresh-baked bread is wafted to the front of the shop to tickle the taste-buds.*
- *Basic essential items (bread, flour, butter, milk, washing powder, etc.) are scattered all over the shop so that you have to pass many displays of other products to find them. Every so often, these essential items are rearranged so that you are forced to re-explore the shop.*
- *Canned music is played at different speeds at different times of the day to control the speed you pass through the shop – special offer announcements are made over the loudspeakers to stimulate interest.*
- *Shelves are always heavily stocked as customers are reluctant to buy from poorly stocked displays.*

Without having to resort to such sophisticated tactics, it is possible to make your displays very effective. Consider the following basic points:

- location;
- size;
- product range;
- lighting and cleanliness;
- enhancing your display.

### Location of displays

People read from left to right, and look from left to right in a new situation, so your display should be placed to the left of the door as they enter the reception area. If possible, locate it in a high traffic area to ensure people see it. One of the best places to have a reception display is near the reception desk. There are several reasons for this:

- Trained staff are immediately on hand to talk to clients and to answer questions.
- Clients may have to wait several minutes to register or to pay which gives them a chance to look at the products.
- Most purchases are made at the time of final payment when the client is leaving.

Product displays can also be located in the consulting room where their main function is to remind personnel to recommend them. However, although they do not need to be large or heavily stocked, some veterinarians feel it puts pressure on a client who is already in a low comfort zone.

Point of sale displays (i.e. products sold from, say, the receptionist's desk at time of final payment) serve to increase sales through impulse purchase. If this technique is used, the goods must be carefully selected to maintain professionalism. There are many items which can be used at point of sale such as rawhide chews, packaged food samples, and bandages, but potentially therapeutic preparations such as vitamin supplements that need explanation to use them properly, or gimmicky toys that detract from the professional image, should be avoided.

> *Another aspect of image is what the client perceives – several Swedish practices I have visited sell dried pig's ears as chews for dogs. Although there is nothing wrong with the concept, how acceptable is this to the caring image of the practice?*

Displays are no use where clients cannot see them. Similarly, they are far less effective where clients cannot pick up and examine the products. Displays behind the reception desk or in glass cabinets are known as museum displays and are not user-friendly.

Practices are increasingly designing separate retail areas off the reception area. As long as they are still readily accessible to the trained reception staff, this has several advantages:

- It helps retain the more clinical and less commercial feel of the reception area.
- It focuses all the products in one area so that they are easier to see.

The problem is people will often not go into these retail areas unless they are specifically looking for something – they are not high traffic areas, which may reduce their profitability.

### Size of display and quantity to stock

The main purpose of a display is to raise client awareness of the products you recommend, so displays do not *have* to be big to increase sales significantly. However, the bigger they are, the more powerful they tend to be.

A guide to the quantity to stock can be obtained fom your wholesaler who should know your potential sales ability. You should be able to order fast-moving items such as foods for healthy pets so that you need to maintain minimum stock (see below, Stock control).

### Choice of products and product range

There is clear guidance for veterinarians about which medicinal products can and cannot be sold from veterinary practices:

> **Sale and Supply of Veterinary Medicinal Products**
> *Medicinal products are classified into three main categories under Part III of the Medicines Act:*
> *General Sales List Medicines (GSLs)*
> *Prescription Only Medicines (POMs)*
> *Pharmacy Medicines (Ps)*
> *A fourth category of importance to veterinary surgeons is the Pharmacy and Merchants List (PML medicines) which includes medicinal products which comes within The Medicines (Veterinary Drugs)(Pharmacy and Merchants List) Order 1989.*
>
> *A veterinarian is able to supply and prescribe medicines in all these categories provided those in the last three categories are 'for administration by him or under his direction to an animal or herd which is under his care'. It is therefore contrary to the provisions of the Act and professionally unethical for a veterinarian to supply products not on the general sale list to any person for administration to an animal or herd which is not under his care.*
> (Legislation Affecting the Veterinary Profession in the United Kingdom, 1993, p. 53)

In addition, even though GSL medicines can be supplied to anyone:

> *All medicines sold or supplied by a veterinarian are by definition 'dispensed medicines' and ... must be labelled ... (according to specified requirements)*
> *Ibid*, p. 59

> *P, PML and GSL may be displayed in waiting rooms, etc. Unless secure cabinets are available, dummy packs should be used for displays of P and PML products. POM medicines should not be advertised or displayed to the public.*
> RCVS Guide to Professional Conduct, 1993, appendix 6.1.10, p. 82

Your veterinary wholesaler should be able to advise you about which are the top-selling brands in any range, and the quantity of each to stock. I do not recommend stocking a wide range of similar products as it confuses clients, and shows that the practice does not have a clear idea about the value of each product.

> *For example, one practice I visited counted seven different types of wormers on their display. Even though they were an equine and small animal practice, they were able to reduce this to four they could confidently recommend.*

Select only those products that you feel confident to use and recommend. Show clients your sincerity by using the products for your own animals.

Talk to colleagues about what they retail in their practices. You don't have to retail different things from your competitors to have good sales – in fact, often sales of a product increase when clients see it in several different outlets.

Listen to what clients are asking for and respond to their needs with top-quality products.

## How to display products on shelves

The following are tips to improve the way you arrange products on your display:

- Shelves should always be full of well-organized, clean products.
- 'Eye level is buy level' and the middle sizes of a product with a range of sizes should be placed at this level.
- Smaller sizes of a product go higher, larger sizes lower on the shelves.
- Don't display damaged or out-of-date products.
- Avoid artistic arrangements of products – they deter purchasers.
- Place life-cycle products from left to right, starting with the young animal on the left.
- Block merchandise vertically as people tend to scan horizontally and this increases the range of products they see.
- Do not use price tags on products, but place them to the right of the product on the shelf. In this way the client sees the product before the price and so is able to appraise the product before finding out how much it costs.
- Displays should always be well stocked: more purchases are made from full shelves than half-empty ones.

Where the traffic flow is from left to right past a particular display unity, the potential 'take-off' of product along the shelves both horizontally and vertically will be in the following proportions (Little, 1992):

| | | | |
|---|---|---|---|
| 4.5% | 2.6% | 2.6% | 5.2% |
| 12.0% | 7.0% | 7.0% | 14.0% |
| 10.5% | 6.0% | 6.0% | 12.3% |
| 3.0% | 1.75% | 1.75% | 3.5% |

In addition, the horizontal bands contribute the following potential 'off-take':

| | |
|---|---|
| Reach level | 15% |
| Sight level | 40% |
| Take level | 35% |
| Stoop level | 10% |

This shows that the first and last vertical columns, and two central horizontal columns are the most effective for location of products. Thus, almost 50% of the selling power is contained in only 25% of the space at sight and take level at either end of the display.

Finally, men tend to select from shoulder height, women from waist height. As most clients to a veterinary practice are women you can position a very powerful display.

### Creating an attractive display

Spot lights or imaginative lighting focus attention on a display and make it more attractive. Careful choice of colour for the shelves and diplay units makes them more inviting. Make sure the shelves are well stocked with products arranged in neat lines, and that the display is clean. No one wants to buy from a grubby display in a dark corner of a room.

A shelf or unit product display can be enhanced by using posters and pictures of normal and unhealthy animals. Posters and models can also be used to create a product focus that links a product with a service, for example, illustrations of fat dogs before and after slimming could enhance the value of a slimming diet.

### Making the display really effective

People use all their senses when they are buying. Make sure your clients are able to do this with your display:

- *Sight*. Make the display visually appealing and clean. Make sure the product name and instructions for use are not obscured by labels.
- *Hearing*. Is this product a spray? A powder? A full can? Damaged?
- *Smell*. How does this product smell?
- *Touch*. What is the weight and texture of this product? What does it feel like?

Displays should be accessible to clients so that they can pick up and handle products. Change them at least every 2 months to create interest in the products. Cross-merchandise products to create a 'package': for example a 'Complete kitten kit' could include a cat basket, starter pack of kitten growth food, basic grooming tools, and a food and water bowl.

## Answer the buying questions

Potential purchasers seek the answers to five questions:

- What is it?
- Why should I buy it?
- How much does it cost?
- Of what use/value is it to me/my pet?
- Should I buy it now?

Answer these using 'shelf-talkers'. These are signs that attach to the front of the shelf and which can increase sales by as much as 300%. Make them easy to read and professional in appearance.

*For example, a shelf-talker for the kitten kit above could be:*

*Complete Kitten Kit.*
*Give your kitten the best start.*
*Get all the things your kitten needs for only £ xxx.*
*Offer applies to the end of the month.*

*For example, for a premium growth diet for puppies:*

*X-brand puppy growth food.*
*Veterinary recommended.*
*Costs yyp/day to feed.*
*Gives your puppy a healthy start.*
*Choose from 2 kg, 5 kg, 10 kg and 20 kg.*

### Using support literature

Product literature and information can be located on or near displays. It is not effective to merely place them in a pile on the display – they should have a proper display box that fits onto the display unit. Leaflets should also be available behind reception for the receptionists to use to support verbal recommendations.

## Calculating the profit from retailing

### To calculate mark-up in per cent:

$$\text{Mark-up } \% = \frac{(\text{selling price} - \text{purchase price})}{\text{purchase price}} \times 100\%$$

e.g. a shampoo bought for 50 p and sold for 75 p has a mark-up of:

$$= \frac{(75 - 50)}{50} \times 100\%$$

$$= 50\%$$

### To calculate profit margin in per cent

$$\text{Profit margin } \% = \frac{(\text{selling price} - \text{purchase price})}{\text{selling price}} \times 100\%$$

e.g. the same shampoo has a profit margin of:

$$= \frac{(75 - 50)}{75} \times 100\%$$

$$= 33.3\%$$

### Pricing and profit margins

The net profit from retailing is calculated by subtracting the costs of staff training, staff time, capital in stock and so on from the income generated by sales of the products. If the income from retailing accounts for less than 15% of the gross income then probably no extra costs are incurred from staff.

If the income from retailing in the practice is more than 15% of the gross then it is better to run the retail business as its own profit centre.

## Pricing for profit

It is recommended to work on *at least* a 33% mark-up to ensure rapid turnover of stock, and keep the practice competitive (compare with a mark-up of a minimum 100% for prescription medicines). Although this may not seem to be a large profit margin, on fast-moving items such as pet foods the profit comes from the repeat sales. Profit margins may be significantly increased where wholesale discounts are obtained.

## Effect of discounting

Underpricing or discounting is risky and unprofitable:

| Price | Mark-up | Units | Profit | Change | Units | Profit |
|-------|---------|-------|--------|--------|-------|--------|
| £1 | 33% | 100 | £33 | | | |
| | | | | −10% | 143 | £33 |
| | | | | +10% | 77 | £33 |

As the example above shows, 43% more product has to be sold to generate the same profit if an item is discounted by 10%. Of course, sometimes it is worth a brief period of discounting as part of a mini-promotion to move or clear out stock, but discounting is often seen as a sign of lack of confidence in a product, and its effect can be to make the practice look like a bargain-basement store.

It is important to remember that in veterinary practice, you are promoting products you believe in and trust, and you are selling them based on their value to the pet, not the price. Clients *want* products they can trust and are prepared to pay for them, so don't be frightened to price profitably.

## Stealing

In some practices, stealing from displays is felt to be a problem. This can be alleviated by using closed displays, or dummy packs (available in some cases from distributors), but these displays also serve to reduce sales effectiveness.

Not infrequently, it is staff who steal either by taking products for personal use directly from stores or displays, or by charging up a false transaction on the cash register. Where this is not part of a staff agreement this can significantly affect profits. It can be controlled by strict stock control and making sure staff order and pay for the items they require.

### Stock turnover

Stock represents capital, and unnecessarily high stocking-levels ties up money and reduces profits. While it is necessary to have adequate stock to supply clients' needs, it is wasteful to overstock, especially if it goes over the product expiry date. Total stock should turnover at least 10 times per year in small animal practice, and at least 6 times per year in large animal practice. Fast-moving retail items such as petfood may turnover far more often than this.

Stock can also take up a lot of space in a practice, especially in those designed before bulky petfoods were so popular. Where space really is a problem, good-sized retail displays can serve as primary storage space.

## Conclusion

Professional retailing offers huge scope for increasing practice revenue. It is estimated that 85% of pet health care purchases are made outside of veterinary practices which means there is tremendous opportunity for the profession to improve their service to their clients.

Ultimately, it is your personal choice whether you want to retail in your practice or not, but as long as you only retail those products which you feel confident recommending and as long as you retail them in a suitably professional manner then they can only benefit the practice.

## Summary

1 Professional retailing is an integral part of excellent client service.

2 Professional retailing is a skill that requires knowledge of which products to buy, how to stock and display them, and how to talk about them to clients.

3 Retailing is profitable because it takes little time, primarily involves support staff and increases the opportunity for other business from clients through increased contact from repeat sales.

# 11 Marketing Your Practice

*Organizations typically become aware of marketing when their market undergoes a change.*

Kotler and Clarke, Business Management Consultants

THE term marketing in relation to veterinary practice often causes a hostile and negative response: 'Professionals don't need to market themselves!'. However, marketing should not scream 'hire me', but must gently suggest, 'here are some sound reasons why you might like to get to know us better'. Marketing plays a major role in the management and development of professional service firms such as veterinary practice, and is an integral part of the successful practice.

Why is marketing not done better in veterinary practices? It is partly through ignorance and lack of awareness of what marketing really entails, but it is primarily because marketing is a *management* issue. Marketing activities represent an *investment* – they require a fair amount of non-money-making time to be spent with uncertain long-term results, and few practices are well-organized enough to manage their investment activities. Although *results* may be recognized and rewarded, the value of marketing *efforts* have to be recognized too – and this requires careful management.

Marketing is surrounded by many myths and misconceptions which colour understanding of what marketing is and what it sets out to achieve:

- *Marketing is advertising and selling.* While advertising and selling are both acceptable marketing communications activities, they represent only a very limited section of the whole marketing function.
- *'We don't 'do' any marketing!.* This concept is linked with the first – that to 'do' marketing you must produce a glossy brochure or have a television advertisement. Marketing is an integral part of having a business and exists at even the most rudimentary level in the logo on the practice notepaper, the clean white coat, and the friendly pat on the head for the dog. It is part of traditional 'bedside manner'. To be really effective, however, marketing activities have to be more explicit and organized.

- *Our senior partner/head nurse/etc. 'does' our marketing!.* Marketing is a lot more than talking to the kennel club annually. Organized marketing is a managerial decision, but marketing happens in the practice all the time – *all* client contact is marketing. Thus, an indifferent receptionist is bad marketing for the practice, whereas the nurse who goes out of the way to help a client is excellent marketing.
- *Marketing means meeting client needs at any cost.* This belief is based on the concept that, 'marketing means giving clients exactly what they want – and all they want is top service for pitiful fees which means we go out of business'. This is *not* what marketing is all about.

## So, what is marketing?

*Marketing is the analysis, planning, implementation and control of carefully formulated programmes which are designed to encourage and build a productive and profitable relationship between an organization, such as a veterinary practice, and its target market, a specific group or groups of animal owners.*

Marketing is a management skill that matches the practice's personnel, resources and expertise with clients' needs in such a way that the practice achieves its long-term goals and the clients receive continued satisfaction. It is not a haphazard process but a specific managerial task that requires carefully formulated plans designed to achieve certain responses. These plans are most effective aimed at specific, target markets and offer what the market wants, not what the practice *thinks* the market wants. To motivate and inform the market well the practice relies heavily on factors such as effective pricing and good communication (see later).

Marketing is essential to ensure the practice's survival and continual health through serving its markets more effectively. It consists of a blend of the 'marketing mix':

- design of the services to be offered (see The problems of marketing services, below);
- pricing (see, Fees and fee-setting, Appendix 1);
- communication/advertising;
- location of the practice.

In this chapter I do not attempt to tell you *how* to market, but explain the background to marketing and why it is import, highlight the common pitfalls with marketing veterinary services and discuss key marketing concepts.

## ■■■ Why do we market?

> *. . . the services veterinarians think their clients don't want most clients won't want. Why? Because they don't know they are available.*
> Don Dooley, Veterinary Management Consultant

The purpose of marketing is three-fold:

- ■ To ensure that current clients stay with the practice.
- ■ To generate more business from the existing client base.
- ■ To attract new clients to use the practice's services.

Although it is possible to achieve these aims without help, I would suggest hiring experienced marketing consultants who can use their training and experience to develop appropriate marketing systems. They will also help you answer the following key questions;

- ■ What is our business? (See Chapter 2, p. 25).
- ■ Who is our client?
- ■ What do they buy?
- ■ What is value to our clients?

### *Who is our client?*

*Which* clients want *your* business? Clients – that is, animal owners – provide your business and it is important to identify who they are. For example, a referral practice may devote a significant part of its marketing efforts towards attracting the support of colleagues in sending them referral cases, whereas to develop a feline speciality a practice would concentrate on marketing its unique services to cat owners.

> *A practice that was setting up a Senior Health Programme decided, as a method of increasing client numbers, to concentrate their marketing efforts on the owners of older pets who had not been into the practice within the last eighteen months. The practice had a zero response and was, needless to say, somewhat disheartened. Unfortunately, these clients are the ones least likely to be interested in their*

*pets' welfare, least likely to want to spend money on their pets, and most likely to be dissatisfied with the practice. Had the practice concentrated on its 'good' clients who want the best for their pets, bring their pet regularly to the practice and who have a good relationship with the practice, they would have had a very different response.*

### What do they buy?

A person buying a microwave oven buys the easiest way to cook food; a person buying a car can buy comfort, safety, transport, or status (or all four). Your clients are actually buying peace of mind when they come to your practice (see Chapter 2, p. 25).

### What is value to our clients?

The traditional answer is price – the true answer is actually far more complex and involves quality and service too (see Chapter 8 and Appendix 1). High price in some situations is actually a value to people, for example buying a fur coat (status) or an expensive perfume (luxury).

## Market to established or new clients?

*Most professional firms say that their existing clients represent the most probable (and often the most profitable) source of new business. However, when one examines their behaviour, one finds that while they have well-established and organized programmes for 'new client' business development, there is little, if any, organized effort to obtain new business from existing clients.*
David Maister, Business Management Consultant

Practices can market to established clients or to attract new clients. However, studies have shown that it is less effective, and five times more costly to market to new clients.

Working with existing and/or new clients requires different approaches. The former is more intimate, more personal and more involved; the latter, being more impersonal, may suit some people better than others. Ideally, practices should aim for a balance between the two. Some of the advantages and disadvantages of marketing to the two different types of clients are highlighted below.

### New business from existing clients

■ Winning client trust and confidence is a major influence in the sales process of veterinary services, which requires an understanding of the client's concerns and needs. It cannot be stressed enough that these needs are not what the *practice* thinks the client wants but what the *client* really wants – which can only be found out by asking the client. Where a good relationship exists with the client, they are more likely to accept the practice's proposal for further care and treatment if a new problem is discovered than to consider the effort of going to a new practice.

■ Marketing costs to win a specific volume of new work from existing clients are much lower than to attract the same volume from new clients.

■ Follow-on treatments for existing clients are often more profitable based on their trust and faith in you, than work gleaned from new clients. For example, an established client is more likely to undertake a senior health check for their pet than a new client.

■ Profitability can be increased, over time, because more work can be done by non-veterinarians as the client learns to trust and accept younger, less experienced staff in the practice.

■ Established clients are more likely to 'give the practice a chance' with something new so that the practice is able to develop and grow its capabilities.

### The importance of winning new clients

■ New clients offer new challenges.

■ They avoid 'overworking' the relationship with established clients.

■ New clients are a long-term marketing investment if the practice has well-established systems for developing business with established clients.

### Client loyalty

Client loyalty is an area of client relations where there is often confusion. A strong sense of allegiance exists with some clients who can be devoted to a particular veterinarian or practice. However, in marketing terms, loyalty means less an attitude than the *behaviour of purchasing the same product repeatedly*. Although the former is desirable for a practice, the latter is the business aim of the practice – to get satisfied clients coming back again and again with their animals.

# ■ The problems of marketing services

Veterinary practice is an example of a professional service industry: it sells professional services to clients to create business. A service is defined as: *any activity or benefit that one party can offer to another that is essentially intangible and does not result in the ownership of anything.* Its production may or may not be tied to a physical product. Thus, a practice does not sell purely a vaccine but a vaccination package of health care (a clinical examination by a qualified animal health care expert, a vaccination which prevents serious diseases, and reassurance for the client that they are doing the right thing for their pet).

## *Features of services*

Services have a number of features that distinguish them from products and which make them more challenging to market. These are:

- *Intangibility* – a service cannot be measured, held in the hand, or tried out before purchase; the buyer has to have faith in the service. This faith comes partly from trust in the person providing the service, but can also be enhanced by making the service as tangible and concrete as possible through describing the benefits of the service, and using specific, descriptive names for the service. Relating the service to the human equivalent may also help people visualize the service. Thus an Annual Pet Dental Health Check is a clinical examination recommended by the veterinarian for your pet every year, to help your pet maintain healthy teeth and gums.
- *Inseparability* – a service cannot exist separately from its providers whether they are persons or machines for example, a vaccination cannot be given without a veterinarian or nurse to do it.
- *Variability* – a service is not only made up of many different parts, its interpretation will vary according to who provides the service. For example, a senior veterinarian may put less emphasis on the value of preventive nutrition than a keen graduate, even though it has been agreed that the service is available from the practice. Similarly, the response to a service may vary according to the owner's interpretation, or the pet's reaction.
- *Perishability* – unlike a product, a service cannot be stored. Much of the content of a service is knowledge, and if the service is not used it is wasted.

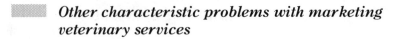

## *Other characteristic problems with marketing veterinary services*

Marketing veterinary services also has a number of other characteristic problems that need to be addressed:

### Third-party accountability

Veterinary practice is subject to third-party accountability which often involves the opinion of other members of the profession. For example, it is not regarded as acceptable to continue dispensing corticosteroids to a patient without regular examination. Sometimes this third-party accountability may involve ethical and legal aspects of the profession, for example perceived cruelty by a veterinary surgeon, or giving treatment to an animal that is not under the practitioner's care.

### Client uncertainty

Clients buying veterinary services are not able to confidently evaluate the services either before or after receiving them, which means they are often uncertain of the *value* of a particular service.

### Does my pet really need this treatment or is the vet simply trying to make money out of me?

Client education is an integral and essential part of veterinary services marketing so that clients can evaluate professional services confidently, understand if and when they should seek veterinary advice, and how to employ the veterinarian productively (see Education of clients, Chapter 5, p. 60; also Chapter 9).

### Experience is essential

Clients seek veterinarians with prior experience of their animal's particular problem. 'Newness' is not a favourable professional characteristic whereas it is often highly desirable with products, for example new flavour, new consistency, new action. New services in a practice are therefore challenging to market because they may require a whole different way of thinking for both the practice and the client.

### Limited differentiability

Differentiating similar services is, unfortunately, not as easy as adding a different sugar coating or flavour to a product. Veterinary services have a limited differentiability from practice to practice – that is, what *is* the difference in having a bitch spayed at practice A compared to practice B? Where a practice is striving to be unique through quality, standards, or the range of services it offers, it needs to market these *differences* very clearly to its clients. This can be done by critically assessing the practice's weaknesses and strengths, then selecting one or two of the strongest characteristics and emphasizing these to clients at every opportunity. How to give the practice a unique and individual 'personality', which is of greater value than the competition in the eyes of potential clients, is one of the greatest challenges facing veterinary practice.

## Maintaining quality control

Veterinary practice is a people organization, run by people for people. As a result, quality control of the services it offers is difficult to standardize because there are so many variables. Not only are there personality and ability differences among the personnel in the practice, but the behaviour of clients and their pets can vary so much too, from the unco-operative owner to the biting dog.

## Making doers into sellers

Most veterinarians are 'doers' – they are trained to do a professional job – they are not sellers. However, before 'buying' veterinary services clients like to meet and become acquainted with the veterinarians and their staff. As a result, veterinarians must learn to 'sell' themselves to be able to sell their services. Many veterinarians do not have the personal characteristics that make them good at selling but can benefit from training in sales and presentation techniques, and from working alongside suitably trained support staff. This training is part of the role of a practice manager.

## Allocating professionals time to marketing

Marketing creates a dilemma – time for a veterinarian means money, but marketing as an activity does not directly generate money (e.g. a talk to the local cat club, or a poster put up in the reception area advertising an obesity clinic). However, it is essential that practice marketing involves the veterinarians because they are the key service providers.

## Pressure to react rather than proact

It is common in practice to be so time-pressurized that all the energy is focused on reacting to clients' demands and there is little or no energy left over for proactively marketing services.

## Effects of advertising are unknown

There is still little known about the effects of advertising professional services. The professions have been long bound by strict rules governing the ethics of advertising. Even though these rules are slowly relaxing, there is a risk of advertising backfiring and being seen as unacceptable. There is a need for clear guidelines like those that exist for advertising non-professional goods and services.

### Limited marketing base knowledge

Little information is available for veterinary practices on the basics of marketing professional services. For historic reasons, marketing is only just becoming acceptable – and perceived as necessary – by all the professions.

## ■■■ Common mistakes

There are four critical but common mistakes that veterinary practitioners make when they start considering marketing for their practices:

- They refuse to employ experienced, professional marketing consultants, believing they can 'do it themselves'.
- They define and limit marketing to 'getting new clients'.
- They misunderstand or refuse to examine the organizational and attitudinal changes necessary in the practice for effective marketing.
- They neglect to tie individual marketing efforts into the practical staff appraisal system, so there is no reward or recognition of individuals' efforts in marketing the practice they work in.

## ■■■ So, how should we market?

So far, I have painted a rather gloomy picture of the problems that beset marketing professional veterinary services. But services can and should be marketed to create a healthy, growing practice and there are various more or less effective ways of doing this.

### *Makeshift marketing approaches*

Where the value of marketing for the benefit of the whole practice is still under debate, makeshift, but generally not very effective, methods of marketing include:

- *Sending key practice members to marketing seminars.* This creates the problem of them returning full of enthusiasm for new ideas and projects but facing the resistance of a practice that has not accepted the necessity for change. As a result, some of the new methods will be tried out in a rather half-hearted way, invariably fail, and then reduce the value of any further, more serious marketing attempts.

■ *Inviting marketing students to research a key aspect of the practice business.* This may create some useful baseline data for the practice, but the students will lack the knowledge and experience of how to use that information effectively in the practice.

■ *Hiring specific marketing agents as needed.* Practice marketing is a management issue that requires constant commitment. It is not something that can be hired out in bits to 'experts'.

■ *Relying on marketing 'packages' and assistance.* e.g vaccination packages These serve mainly to raise awareness of marketing possibilities. They do not affect the whole practice's attitude to total marketing. Again, marketing in bits is not effective.

## Effective marketing

Effective marketing is about showing selected clients that you can satisfy their needs. It requires careful planning, and the involvement and support of everyone in the practice, especially the practice principal(s). In addition, staff in the practice must understand the *value* and *benefits* of marketing.

### *What services does the practice offer?*

Start by establishing the services the practice has to offer. This includes everything from having well-trained, friendly staff to a good parking area; from ultrasonography facilities to obesity counselling; from a 24-hour emergency service to a vaccination programme. It is not necessary at this stage to increase the range of services, rather concentrate on doing better with the ones you have.

### *What do our clients want?*

The only way to find out what clients want of you is to ask them. Short, focused questionnaires for clients about particular services can be invaluable (see Appendix 3).

## What is the competition and how do we differentiate ourselves from it?

Competition is not something to be frightened of. Competition, both from other veterinary practices and pet-related businesses, can have a very positive effect on business. For example, practices selling premium quality petfoods for healthy pets often find their sales are *increased* when another source starts selling the same food locally, because a wider client base see the food, and are not so suspicious of it being a 'Vets Only' product.

Carefully selected services that differentiate the practice can be very wide-based. For example, they might include:

- convenient location;
- long opening times;
- hiring top-quality, client-centred staff;
- small animal/feline/exotic specialization;
- specialist referral component;
- total pet health care programmes.

## Market the benefits: ask the 'So what?' question

Services are sold on the benefits they offer the client and their pet. To identify the benefits of a service ask yourself the 'So what?' question (see also Chapter 10, p. 135, Selling professional products).

| Service | SO WHAT? | Benefit |
|---|---|---|
| Large car park | | Easy parking for our clients |
| Friendly, well-trained staff | | Willing and helpful in providing care information specific to your pet |
| Radiography facilities | | Useful and rapid aid to diagnosis so that we can start treating your pet more quickly and accurately |
| Ophthalmology specialist service | | To better help you, the client, and your pet in an environment you are familiar and happy in |

### Internal marketing to staff

Marketing to every member of the staff is an ongoing and essential component of the whole marketing programme. Reinforce the value of marketing to staff as part of the growth and development, and ongoing success of the practice.

### Attention to detail

Marketing is a specialized form of communication. When you market your practice you are *communicating* it to your clients – you are *communicating* the values, services and professional products you recommend in the practice.

Communication involves all of the senses, especially sight, hearing, smell and touch. Think carefully about how each of these applies to how you market your practice:

> *For example, the outside of the practice:*
> *Does it* look *clean and smart?*
> *Can clients* hear *animals in the kennels crying when they are out in the street?*
> *Can they* smell *the practice, or see the dog faeces in the car park?*

> *For example, the reception area:*
> *Does it* look *professional, friendly, and clean?*
> *Can the client* hear *the staff joking and time-wasting on the telephone whilst waiting for an appointment?*
> *Is the receptionist wearing an overpowering perfume?*
> *Do the magazines* feel *clean?*

> *For example, having a consultation:*
> *Does the veterinarian* look *professional and competent?*
> *Can the client* hear *animals crying and howling in another part of the building?*
> *Does the room* smell *of anal glands from a previous consultation?*
> *Is the room clean and fresh, or does everything* feel *grubby and* look *worn?*

## Communication tools for marketing veterinary practice

Figure 11.1 illustrates some of the communication tools available to veterinary practices to market their services. When instigating any of the

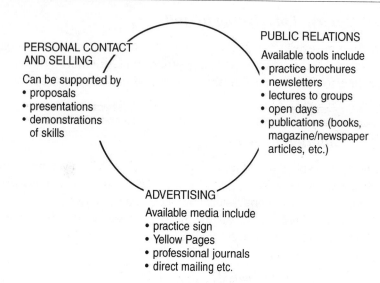

**Figure 11.1** *Some examples of the communication tools available for marketing veterinary practice.*

methods listed it is important to establish a system to measure their effect, such as incorporating a response element in a practice newsletter, or counting the number of referral cases from colleagues that result from advertising in professional journals.

A common mistake made by veterinary practices is to judge the effect of a promotion simply on 'gut feelings'. For example many practices claim they sell 'loads' of a certain product or product range that they are promoting, when, in actual fact, they have no hard data on the sales figures, and are often shocked to find how little they sell in reality when compared to other practices with organized campaigns. It is important not to rely on personal evaluation or intuition. The veterinarian is not part of the target audience and therefore their opinion is of little worth in this situation.

## Advertising

Advertising is a specialized form of communication. Specific examples of 'pure' advertising are Yellow Pages advertisements and the sign outside the practice. Although the veterinary profession is still ethically restricted in what exact form advertising can take, a practice constantly advertises itself. The appearance and behaviour of the staff, the appearance of the building, even the appearance and quality of the stationery used by the practice advertise the standards in the practice.

### Personal selling

Personal selling of services is a powerful and effective communication method used to create business by establishing a personal relationship with a group or organization such as kennel/cattery owners, breeders, farmers looking for herd health schemes, etc. To attract referral work from colleagues, personal demonstration of skills coupled with lectures and seminars is often the most effective way of communicating the services available. The various stages are shown in Fig. 11.2 and are based on attracting the client, and building and maintaining an ongoing relationship with them.

### Public relations

Public relations take many forms from sending out a friendly and informative practice newsletter, to being the popular local practice reported by the local newspaper for helping rescue the old lady's cat from a tree. Lectures to interested groups of animal owners can be good public relations, or can seek to create business, for example outlining the benefits of a flock health scheme to a group of sheep farmers.

The practice identity is established through public relations which includes all the literature that the practice produces (see Appendix 3, Use of practice literature). Careful consideration of the practice logo, and having professional help with brochure and newsletter production are investments that are well worth making.

## Marketing and quality

Many practices claim to offer high-quality service based on the fact that they employ technically highly competent staff, and are exceptionally well

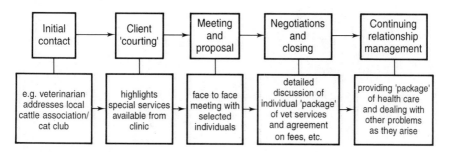

**Fig. 11.2** *The personal selling process.*

equipped with all the latest diagnostic and therapeutic gadgets. However, this is only part, and probably the least important part of professional service quality.

Quality, its exact definition, and its control and measurement are discussed in considerable detail in Chapter 8. In simplest terms, *perceived quality* is the difference between a client's *expectations* of a veterinary service, and how the client *perceives* that the particular service lived up to those expectations.

A practice that is serious about its commitment to quality will systematically measure quality perceptions. Quality is the key to differentiation of practices.

## ▆▆▆ Summary ▆▆▆

1   Marketing is the analysis, planning, implementation and control of carefully formulated programmes designed to bring about voluntary exchanges of values with target markets for the purpose of achieving organizational objectives.

2   Its purpose is to grow the practice's business.

3   Marketing involves everybody in the practice, and is constant and ongoing.

4   Marketing in veterinary practice presents particular problems because the 'products' being marketed are services, that are intangible and cannot be owned.

5   To overcome this, identify the features and market the benefits of services in practice.

# 12 Looking to the Future

*The most significant challenge facing the veterinary profession today is not competition or recession, but rather our own ability to change the habits that got us where we are today.*

Thomas Catanzaro, Veterinary Management Consultant

THE only constant feature of today's business world is change. Change by its very nature is not static: we constantly face new challenges. I believe the most important challenge we face is ourselves, the veterinary profession. Change will continue to go on around us all the time – we need to review *our* ability and willingness to respond to change.

Veterinarians are highly trained, intelligent and generally ambitious people. More and more are becoming dissatisfied and disillusioned about life in practice. This disillusionment starts early – more than 15% of young graduates interviewed in the SPVS survey in 1992 were not content with practice. There is a steady drift from practice to other branches of the profession or even out of the profession altogether. Why is this happening?

> *If today's young professionals appear less motivated than in the past, it is not because they cannot be motivated. Rather it is because the source of motivation that existed in the past, and the mechanisms through which they worked, are no longer as forceful or effective as they were.*
> David Maister, Business Management Consultant

In this chapter some of the problems the profession is currently facing are identified and some solutions are offered.

## 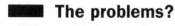 The problems?

### 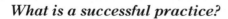 *What is a successful practice?*

'Success' is a rather subjective term. In an attempt to define it, 'successful' practices (identified by colleagues and others associated with the profession) were evaluated on a number of criteria (see Table 12.1). The successful practices outperformed average practices in every one. They performed outstandingly well financially, practised high-quality medicine, had high levels of client satisfaction, and the practice principals felt they had an excellent quality of life (unpublished report, courtesy of Hills Pet Nutrition, Inc.). These results show that practice is far more than helping sick animals.

## The selection process of students

There is much debate about student selection – and no simple answer. A veterinary education undoubtedly requires students who are capable of studying long, hard hours – but these are not the characteristics then needed in the field. Having a prerequisite period of working on farms, at riding stables and helping in practices before acceptance into university may help screen out some of the more unsuitable potential applicants, but still seems to admit youngsters with a very idealized view of what is involved in being a practising veterinarian.

**Table 12.1** *Criteria for comparison*

Eight general criteria for practice success were examined in 54 North American veterinary hospitals that had been selected by colleagues, practice management consultants and others as being outstandingly successful practices. These practices completed a very detailed questionnaire which revealed that they were very different from national averages in every category.

- **Practice mission:** over 80% shared a common vision and had stated goals
- **Personnel management:** over 90% supported/provided further education for support and professional staff
- **Client service:** over 95% offered medical recalls and client education programmes, and all provided a range of preventive health care programmes
- **Quality of medicine and surgery:** over 80% felt they aggressively sought to learn and implement new procedures, equipment and products
- **Community and professional involvement:** over 80% were active in different ways in the community
- **Practice growth:** over 80% had used a practice management consultant, and all had a multi-user computer system
- **Quality of personal and professional life:** nearly 100% felt they had an excellent quality of personal and professional life
- **Financial performance:** average transaction fees, profit per veterinarian, and other financial parameters were all higher than the national average

(Unpublished report, courtesy of Hills Pet Nutrition, Inc., 1994)

### Poor university preparation for life in practice

University education is, naturally, very academic, which is not adequate preparation for the more physical demands of life in practice. In addition, there is still little or no training in the extremely important areas of good communication, client relations and business management.

### Poorly established support and training systems for the new graduate in practice

The experiences of some new graduates in practice are not good: unsympathetic, unsupportive bosses; fierce support staff; overwhelming work schedules; loneliness; low standard accommodation; and rude animal owners, to name but a few problems. Over four-fifths of British graduates go into general practice. Less than half of them receive job training on routine procedures such as the vaccination regimen in the practice, routine surgical procedures, and sales of drugs and diets (Hill, 1993). Graduates are often left to fend for themselves which not only can create problems in the practice, but also can lower their often already fairly low self-confidence.

### Poor salaries, especially at graduate level

Veterinary graduates today suffer the effects of frozen student grants – they leave college with a millstone of student loans around their neck. After 5 years of intensive education and training, British graduates then look forward to salaries that start at around £13 000 p.a. (the minimum is £10 000) For which they are expected to work exceedingly long, unsocial hours pay their living expenses *and* pay back the loans.

In comparison with other health care professions, the veterinary profession is the worst compensated financially. This is a sad reflection of the confidence felt by a self-financing profession in their professional skills and abilities (see also Chapter 2, p. 16).

### No career structure

What can a vet do to progress both professionally and personally after 5 years, 10 years, 20 years in practice? The problem of the mature, experienced assistant and how to treat them is increasing – especially as more and more veterinarians (particularly women) are opting not to buy into partnerships.

## A partnership is not a career move

Setting up your own plate or becoming a partner by buying into a practice was often seen as the ultimate goal for a veterinary surgeon. Today's graduates see this neither as a career move (in fact, it is actually a business rather than a career move) nor a wise investment. Partners are often financially worse off than assistants, and are required to make heavy sacrifices to quality of personal and family life, work excessive and unsocial hours, and commit themselves to one geographic location for an indefinite but usually long period of time. In addition, partnerships can be harrowing to live with and almost impossible to leave.

## *Little support for and encouragement of further education and self-development in practices*

Few practices have a clear idea of what they wish to achieve with further education of staff so CPD efforts tend to be erratic and unstructured. It is often up to the individual – if they have the time and the energy (and the money).

## *Women are fully accepted by the profession yet it continues to 'cold-shoulder' this skilled and highly competent majority section of the workforce*

Women are not men! Women have different needs from men. They tend not to want the traditional 'full time' job of older colleagues. They want more flexibility to be able to combine their professional and personal/family lives.

### Women and partnerships

Many women do not want partnerships. As women form the bulk of the graduating workforce this creates the situation that expensive practices have to be financed with less and less capital input. Not only does this have implications on practice standards, it also has implications for women veterinarians in a profession where significant decisions, political, financial, perhaps even clinical, are traditionally taken by those with capital at stake (SPVS, unpublished survey, 1994).

## *Stress management*

Stress arises when expectations (of self performance) do not meet or are unable to meet reality. This creates guilt, one of the major causes of stress.

Veterinarians tend to be goal-oriented achievers who are overly self-critical and inclined to experience a high sense of personal failure and guilt when they don't meet expected standards of performance.

The profession provides no training in how to recognize and deal with stress. Left to fester, it leads to disillusionment, 'burn-out' and even death. The veterinary profession has the highest suicide rate of all the professions. Is it surprising when one considers the dichotomies veterinarians are constantly up against? (see Table 12.2).

### *Loss of motivation*

*Rarely have I heard of young professionals becoming demotivated because of too much work – most often (all too often) demotivation results from too much **meaningless** work. And since almost no work done by a professional firm is in fact meaningless (it is all, or should be, valuable to clients), this syndrome represents a failure of management.*

David Maister, Business Management Consultant

## Some solutions

### *Look for ideas outside the veterinary profession*

Valuable lessons and insights can be gained through comparison of the veterinary industry with other similar health industries. In a recent North

**Table 12.2** *Some daily stressors*

- Striving for high ideals vs. work devalued by 'It's only an animal'
- Loneliness and exhaustion vs. tendency to overcommit self
- Highly self-critical vs. always feel guilty when something goes wrong
- Veterinarians are 'people-pleasers' vs. feeling of not being appreciated by clients/colleagues
- Highly skilled and very able vs. the client who will not/cannot pay for treatment
- Deep desire to help animals (and their owners) vs. business finance, difficult clients
- Caring for animals (and their owners) vs. frequent exposure to death and grief
- Consider self indispensible and have an obsession with work vs. can't put mistakes in perspective

American survey, the pharmaceutical, dental and ophthalmic industries were compared with veterinary practice on a wide range of parameters including requirements for professional qualification, CPD requirements, professional incomes, support staff incomes, starting salaries for professionals, number of graduates, number of applicants per job/position, etc.

The ophthalmic profession, for example, gave valuable insight into how to handle competition from chain superstores – the ophthalmic equivalent of pet superstores. By listening carefully to their clients' demands and then working to satisfy them, ophthalmists were able to respond successfully to the challenge of a wide range of cheap glasses, immediately, by providing thorough eye examinations, faster service, a larger and better selection of fashionable frames, greater convenience, and better merchandizing (see also below, Changing the staff structure).

The survey concluded that the veterinary profession was not as unique as it thought and that many useful parallels could be drawn with other health professions. It also pointed out that the *impetus for change within the selected industries were their own dynamic professional organizations* (unpublished data, Courtesy of Hills' Pet Nutrition, Inc.).

### The undergraduate syllabus should include communication skills, grief and stress management

Communication skills are essential to success in practice. They are needed to provide a harmonious work environment, and develop the trust relationship with clients that creates business. Undergraduates would benefit enormously from learning skills such as self-presentation, active listening and better telephone manner (see Chapters 4 and 5).

Grief associated with the death of an animal is often as traumatic for the veterinarian as for the owner. It can recall incidences of personal, unresolved grief for the veterinarian, represent failure of a treatment protocol, or simply be the loss of a loved patient. Learning how to help the grieving client, and come to terms with one's own grief is an important part of stress management. Several North American universities and teaching hospitals have now established grief management programmes in their undergraduate syllabus.

Teaching veterinarians to understand the importance of stress, their high predisposition to stress, how to recognize it and how to manage it would go a long way towards reducing the incidence of unhappy and disillusioned practitioners. In the UK, the Veterinary Helpline, a 24-hour telephone service available to veterinarians, provides help and a 'listening ear' in a crisis (see Table 12.3).

**Table 12.3** *The Veterinary Helpline*

The Veterinary Helpline is a 24-hour telephone helpline for veterinarians, registered veterinary practitioners, their spouses and other dependent relatives. Voluntarily manned by members of the profession and their spouses, it aims to provide help and advice on personal problems. It is financed by the Royal College of Veterinary Surgeons and the British Veterinary Association.

**Telephone: 01941 – 170000**

## Business management for undergraduates

Undergraduates should leave university with a basic understanding of business management skills. Veterinary practice is a small business and needs to be run like one to be really successful. Naturally, not all graduates will want to run their own practices, but they would understand and be more inclined to accept the value of hiring a good manager.

## More postgraduate supervised time in recognized teaching practices

Graduates typically lack practical, communication and business skills when they leave university. A system of 'protected learning' for graduates, similar to the human GP training system, in veterinary practices of a defined standard, for a minimum of, say, 2 years before they can be regarded as fully qualified veterinarians would better prepare them for practice life.

Practices would probably require some sort of incentive to employ and train new graduates who, naturally, are not as efficient and productive as more experienced veterinarians. Scholarships might be made available from the pharmaceutical and animal nutrition industries, for example.

## Continuing professional development

In an attempt to co-ordinate and improve practice efforts with CPD, the RCVS Education Trust has part-funded a pilot in practice competition in the north of England (see Table 12.4). Thirty practices are taking part. It will be interesting to see the outcome of this exciting venture.

The option to improve communication skills, learn about grief and stress management, and basic business skills should also be available for practitioners. There is often too much emphasis on clinical matters *if at the*

**Table 12.4** *Aims of Charter 150 CPD in Practice Competition*

- To formalize the organization of CPD within the practice, to work towards achieving individual, practice and professional goals for all members of the practice
- To develop methods of evaluating CPD and improving the application and sharing of knowledge within the practice
- To demonstrate the benefits of investing in planned CPD
- To identify practices who successfully apply systematic techniques and use them as examples to others of what can be achieved

*same time* practitioners are also expected to run their own practices well. I would suggest that the true solution is to encourage practitioners to 'let go' and accept that management of their practices is the job of trained practice managers.

### Create a career structure in practices

It would be quite possible to create a more formalized career structure for practitioners with a range of predetermined salary increases dependent on experience, evidence of attendance at CPD course, and further certification and qualification. Of course, the salary increases would have to be good enough to provide the incentive for further study.

This would require revision of the current rather lackadaisical financial systems of income generation and monitoring present in many practices. For example, individual goal achievement and performance assessments would have to play a far greater role in practice (see Chapter 7).

### Meaningless work?: change the staffing structure

Other professions have learnt the value of leveraging their staff to improve service and profitability. The dental profession is an example of a health care profession that uses support staff in a similar way to the veterinary profession. However, North American dental hygienists are not only paid a lot more than veterinary assistants, they are also given more responsibility and create a significant income for the practice.

In addition, the ratio of support to professional staff is double that in veterinary practices – the dental profession has learnt to make the most of their support staff, leaving professionals to provide the skilled services (that produce the higher revenue). Education, training and increased empowerment of support staff is a key to success in other health industries. Let's do it for the veterinary profession.

Similarly, employing a qualified practice manager would free the practice principals for more profitable work, and enhance professional and support staff productivity.

## More flexible work schedules in practice

Practices need to be more imaginative and flexible with their work schedules to cater for the changing needs of the veterinary workforce. Well over half of all graduates are women. Flexible work schedules enable them to, for example, balance raising a family with continuing in practice or studying further. Of course, these flexible schedules would apply equally well to men.

An example of what is possible can be found in Sweden. Women (or their partners) can take salaried leave from their workplace for up to 2 years to care for their children. Their job is held open until their return. For those who go back to work, excellent local day-care centres that take children from 2 months old are available to everyone. Schools provide after-school care until 6 p.m. for children up to 11 years old. Need this be only a dream in Britain?

## Revision of the 24-hour care obligation

Veterinarians in Britain are required to provide 24-hour service for sick animals. This puts unsocial, unnecessary and unacceptable demands on the modern veterinarian. Local emergency/night clinics which are manned in the unsocial hours would provide high standards of 'out of hours' care as well as relief for practices which function during normal working hours.

## Lay ownership of practices?

The loss of capital investment into practices due to the reluctance of graduates to buy partnerships could be allayed by allowing non-veterinarian ownership of practices (see Chapter 3, p. 32). As long as practices followed certain clearly defined ethical and behavioural guidelines, I believe lay ownership could be a positive injection of fresh ideas and business concepts into today's practices.

# ■■■ Conclusion

The story is not all doom and gloom! The veterinary profession is a fine profession full of dedicated, hardworking individuals with a mass of resources and ideas. Now is the time to become more open-minded and receptive to new ideas, to look outwards to other successful businesses to see how they tackle change, and to boldly face new challenges. Change is something to be excited about. It offers chances to try new things, to be creative, and to develop.

Let's learn *not* be afraid of change. Let's learn to *keep* the bright youngsters who are attracted into the profession. The veterinary profession is a profession to be proud of. Let's make sure it stays that way!

*Appendix 1*

# Setting Fees in Practice

## ■■■ Financial planning

The purpose of financial planning is to take control of the financial development of the practice to create the practice of your vision. At its most simplistic level financial planning consists of:

- deciding on the profit you would like to generate;
- calculating the costs in the practice;
- calculating the income necessary to cover the costs and generate the profit you want.

Outgoings (costs) include staff salaries, heating/lighting/maintenance costs, drug and other stock items, food and accessories, property rates, taxes and insurance, and so on.

Income is generated from professional fees and the sale of professional goods and medicines. It is influenced by the level of professional fees set in the practice, the number of cases seen, and the amount of goods and medicines sold.

Fee-setting is a controversial issue but if is an important part of the healthy, positive attitude of the responsive practice. Although it is beyond the scope of this book to look in any more detail at financial planning for veterinary practice the issue of fee-setting is examined in more detail.

## ■■■ Fee-setting

Clients are more fee sensitive than they used to be, which does not mean they automatically seek the lowest fees. Careful attention to fee-setting can bring substantial returns to a practice, helping to attract clients away from other practices, and to obtain clients who might otherwise have avoided a particular service because they feared it would cost too much.

Fee-setting involves multiple considerations:

- What are the objectives of fee-setting?
- What strategies are available?

- What are the tactics for implementing fee-setting?
- How should fees be changed and how often?
- How can fees be negotiated, invoiced, and collected most effectively?
- Identifying and eliminating the emotional clouding factors to fee-setting.

# ■■■■ Determining the objectives of fee-setting

### ■■ *Practice life-cycle*

The objectives of fee-setting depend on what the practice wants to achieve with its fees and where it is in the practice life-cycle (see Chapter 2). Thus the 'expert' practice will set high fees but expect relatively few clients, whereas the efficient practice will set lower fees but anticipate a high client throughput.

### ■■ *Market penetration*

A practice may want to penetrate a particular market and therefore needs to make itself distinctly different from the competition. For example, a practice may find low fees advisable initially if:

- The market appears to be highly sensitive to fee levels, and therefore a low fee will stimulate a more rapid market growth.
- A low fee would discourage actual and potential competition.
- A low fee would not be viewed by clients as an indicator of poor quality work.

However, if none of these conditions applies then fee-cutting would not be the technique to use, and other methods of market penetration or other objectives should be found.

For most veterinarians, their main objective in fee-setting is to charge a fee that is fair and enables them to cover their time and expenses, and generate a profit that allows them a comfortable (but not extravagant) standard of living. Their reputation as being fair and competent matters more than making lots of money.

### ■■ *Strategic options*

There are two key elements to a fee strategy:

- the average fee level;
- the fee presentation approach.

The practice needs to decide how low or high it wants its fees to be, on average, in comparison to other practices, and how it will present these fees to the client.

There are three basic techniques for determining the average fee level:

■ calculating the cost per procedure;
■ demand-orientated method;
■ competition-orientated method.

The cost per procedure is often a good base to begin from in fee-setting and can be used to create price lists of procedures, and the price of drugs and disposables. These are then combined in different ways for different cases to produce the final fee.

Demand-driven fees are primarily those where clients can fairly easily 'shop around', for example, the cost of vaccinations, neutering, worming, basic examination. They are also routine, common procedures which therefore have relatively fixed overheads.

Competition-determined fees are calculated in relation to neighbouring practices and their charges. There may be a deliberate decision to set fees above or below those of the competition.

In reality, a mixture of all three is used so that, for example, in calculating the fee for a routine procedure such as a bitch spay, the fee to the client would be lower than, say, surgery for a gastric torsion. This is because a spay is a common operation that is relatively standard, is often presented as a fee package (the total cost of a bitch spay including intravenous fluids, pre-and post-op care is £x) and one that clients will phone around practices to get price quotations on. A gastric torsion is not routine, not standard and cannot easily be 'packaged' because it is highly individualized.

### Selecting a fee-presentation approach

In veterinary practice there are three main methods of fee presentation:

■ time and costs;
■ fixed sum;
■ mixture of the two methods.

Fees that are calculated on the basis of the time and costs involved are variable and often more profitable than those routine procedures that have a fixed fee. This is because they reflect the true time and costs involved rather than an estimated average, or the down-valuation of a demand-driven fee.

One major disadvantages of the time and costs approach is the uncertainty and consequent dissatisfaction it creates in clients. The client must make a decision based only on an estimate (provided by the professional) of the total cost of the procedure. Misunderstandings over what a procedure will cost is one of the most common communication problems that arises in practice (see Preventing bad debtors, below).

Another major disadvantage is the tendency of veterinarians to 'shave' the bill to reduce it to a level that they *personally* find acceptable. This is done by 'forgetting' to charge for minor procedures, and disposables. This can represent huge losses to the practice (see Identifying and eliminating the emotional clouding factors, below).

The fixed sum method alleviates client uncertainty over fees and can also be used to 'hide' high hourly/daily rates that clients may have difficulty accepting (as they do not earn these amounts). On the other hand, the procedures can create a lower profit margin and there must therefore be a constant drive to ensure the volume of work that will create the profit.

In practice, a mixture of the two methods is generally used. Fixed sum fees are used for the 'shop around' procedures whereas the time and costs method is used to calculate individual, less routine procedures.

### Tactics for fee-setting

The offering of discounts to clients is common in veterinary practice. It is usually done for clients who:

- require services in a 'slow' or quiet period of the year;
- have a large number of pets and buy a large volume of services;
- need the services to support an animal charity or trust.

Carefully used, it can be a very powerful method of cementing the trust bond with a favoured client. Wrongly used it loses profit and implies the practice charges too high fees anyway.

Another common tactic is the 'high estimate'. Estimating a fee then adding a factor of 25 – 50% serves two functions:

- if the estimate was, in fact, too low there is already an in-built safety factor and the final fee is not a surprise to the client;
- if the estimate was accurate, the client has the bonus of a pleasant surprise.

Referral and second opinion fees should always be higher than ordinary fees. Clients seek professional expertise: this should be charged for accordingly.

## Initiating changes in fees

Whatever the fee policy chosen it is always necessary after a period to change fees to account for inflation, costs, demand for services and competitive factors. The fee change can be general or specific. It is sometimes an advantage to use selective fee changes so that the most sensitive items (the 'shop around' procedures) have little or no alteration in price.

There is always a fear associated with increasing fees that clients will be frightened off and business will decrease. This can be managed in a number of ways:

- having frequent small increases in fees (1/2 – 2% every two months) so that it is difficult to spot increases. This also has the added advantage that it keeps the fees on a level with inflation;
- changing the fees at the time when the maximum level of work is anticipated such as in the summer;
- ensuring staff are informed about fee changes;
- monitoring client response to the fee changes – it is said that if less than 5% of clients complain about your fees they are probably too low!

The effect fee changes will have on clients is extremely difficult to measure. People tend to ignore or avoid information about fees prior to the purchase of a service, paying most attention to this information after the services have been received. This is classically seen when an emergency patient is rushed in and the distraught client will 'pay anything' for treatment, only to complain later that the bill is too high. People are prepared to pay high fees for professionals with outstanding reputations. Fees are an important part of the development of the trust bond with the client, and may be more significant in deciding whether or not the client will *return* to a practice than for making the initial visit. Fees are also a measure of quality of service expected by a client.

The fee structure can change as part of the long-term development plans of the practice. Thus a relatively low-price new practice may become the most expensive practice in the area as their style changes, and their client-base stabilizes.

## Fee communication and collection

The most important point to bear in mind when collecting fees is to *avoid negative surprises*. Careful preparation of a fee estimate which the client sees and accepts, updating the client if there are any changes in the original estimate, and breaking down the final bill into its component pieces can help make the process of fee collection be as painless as possible.

## Itemizing

Itemizing all the procedures carried out on the final invoice has both advantages and disadvantages. On the one hand it educates and informs the client about what was done to the animal, and helps create trust with the practice because nothing is hidden.

On the other hand, itemizing gives more room for client query.

## Preventing bad debtors

It is important to have an established, effective policy for fee collection to avoid bad debts. Such a policy could include some or all of the following:

- For procedures over a certain value, clients sign written estimates to indicate agreement with and acceptance of the costs involved. The client is kept fully informed of any changes in the estimate and may be required to sign new estimates.
- A portion of the costs are paid before the procedure is performed. This is an especially sensible policy in areas where client creditworthiness is dubious.
- When clients join a practice they are required to complete a personal history form that includes details of their bank and credit cards.
- Make payment by major credit cards possible.

Bad debts are not the only way money is lost from fees in practice. Probably the most important way in most practices is through improper charging i.e. missing services and procedures that have been performed.

## Identifying and eliminating the emotional clouding factors

Veterinarians, like many in the caring profession are heavily influenced by emotional factors in relation to fees and fee-setting. Some of these factors are:

- a low self-value based on setting extremely high professional standards for themselves;
- a fear of money: money is not something professional people need to talk about;

- personal ethics;
- need for money;
- fear of client perceptions;
- inability to attach a real value to a service;
- an in-built, fixed, personal ceiling that influences all other decisions.

Support staff are not immune to these clouding factors either. It is an important part of successful practice policy to teach staff how to talk about fees to clients. They should be able to talk confidently not apologetically about fees, be knowledgeable about how a fee is calculated and be able to handle objections to fees without embarrassment.

Computers play an invaluable role in fee calculation and collection. Not only can they generate and alter the price list as necessary, but they can also act as the passive 'third person' when it comes to charging ('The computer says it costs . . .') which can take pressure off staff.

It is very important that clients feel they get value for money. If the practice is to charge the highest fees in town, clients must feel they get the best service from that practice (see Chapter 8). Remember, fees are the clients' view of the value of service they receive.

*Appendix 2*

# Practice Promotional Literature

Practice promotional literature is all of the papers or documents that you produce in the practice for client or business use. It promotes or represents the practice and is one of the many methods of communication used in practice. It is very important to produce literature of a high standard that reflects the professional standards in the practice.

It is worth seeking professional help to design the literature for your practice. Home-produced literature can lack professional finish and quality. Commercial advertising firms often give very reasonable quotations for logo-design, production and printing costs and can give invaluable advice about paper quality, type-style, etc. They are often a significant time-saver for the practice as well.

The following is a brief summary of all the different types of practice promotional literature available with notes on aims and effective presentation of each.

## Client information sheets

*Function:* to give clear, specific instructions/information in simple terms about disease management or pet care.

- To give the owner more understanding of particular health problems.
- To give owner advice on home care.
- To give answers to common questions.
- To inform owners of the benefits of new or existing services/ products in the practice to the benefit of themselves and their pet.

Information sheets can be personalized with the client's and the pet's name and with information specific to their particular problem (if the practice has a computer).

### *Examples of topics suitable for handouts*

- neutering;

- vaccination;
- giving medication – eardrops, eyedrops, pills;
- pre- and post-general anaesthetic care;
- managing surgical drains/bandages/sutures;
- prevention of dental disease;
- the importance of home dental care;
- internal and external parasite control;
- obesity management;
- senior health;
- new puppy/kitten care;
- specific diseases – renal failure, diabetes mellitus, diarrhoea and vomiting, liver failure, etc.;
- emergency care/first aid;
- euthanasia and grief counselling;
- nutrition;
- dealing with common behaviour problems.

### *How to use handouts*

- Fewer than 15% of clients will read a handout if it is just taken from the rack.
- More than 85% will read it if they are handed the leaflet with the words; 'This is important information (about the health of your pet): you should take time to read it. Please feel free to ask us any questions you may have'.
- Include appropriate leaflets in an information pack, for example a puppy pack could include leaflets on nutrition, vaccination, worming, neutering, pet insurance, and the facilities in the practice.
- Provide an appropriate leaflet explaining the use and value of the product when a particular product is purchased, for example diets, shampoos, parasiticides.
- Mail to selected clients.
- Use leaflets as part of a product display.

## Newsletters

*Function:* to inform and update clients with new information of benefit to themselves and their pets. They are particularly useful to market the benefits of owning healthy animals.

A newsletter could contain some of the following:

- seasonal information – fleas, fireworks, heatstroke, hot cars, grass seeds, hair shedding;
- practice specific information – new staff, new services;
- preventive health care information about different programmes, for example dental, obesity, vaccination, senior, puppy care, behaviour;
- ongoing series, for example caring for your kitten, cats of the world;
- interesting cases – to demonstrate challenges in practice and practice facilities;
- client question and answer page;
- 'client corner' with photos of the owners and their pets;
- forthcoming events, for example an open day, National Pet Week.

*Advantages:*

- excellent concept;
- can be mailed to every client, handed out in the practice, used at meetings, etc.;
- often can be partly or wholly sponsored by veterinary companies in return for advertising;
- may have outside authors contributing, local photographers, etc. at no extra cost;
- can be successfully organized and run by a member of the support staff.

*Disadvantages:*

- may be difficult to find the time and motivation to keep producing;
- can be costly – printing, mailing, time;
- not always easy to measure the impact, for example increased uptake of services;
- can you be sure people read them?

## ■■■ Practice brochure

*Function:* to encourage clients to use the practice by describing the practice and all the services it offers in terms of the quality of care and the benefits that the client and their pets receive.

*Consider:*

- cost of production – what is your budget?
- how will you measure the impact on your clients?
- size, appearance, paper quality and colour, contents, message,

number of pages, glossy/matt, photos/illustrations, logo, number to print, how soon out of date? full colour/some colour/black and white?

*To include:*

- front/back page – practice logo, practice details, map;
- practice mission statement;
- number and qualifications of staff;
- specialist/referral facilities;
- major services in the practice expressed in terms of benefits to the client and their pets, for example X-ray, ECG, laboratory, anaesthetics facilities, diathermy, cattery, kennels, operating theatre(s), dental facilities, reception, isolation ward, qualified veterinary nurse care;
- appointment system/open surgeries;
- payment policies.

It is tempting to produce a high quality, full colour, glossy brochure but this will be extremely expensive. Smaller, less glossy productions can be just as effective but with a big cost saving.

### How to use a client brochure

- give to new clients on first visit;
- give several brochures to referring clients;
- send brochures with statements and reminder cards;
- mail brochures to all clients in an area when the practice first opens;
- display in reception and exam room;
- give brochures to prospective clients via family and friends;
- give out brochures when lecturing;
- hand out on open day.

## Reminders

*Function:* to remind clients a service or health check is due, for example dental, vaccination, senior check, pet health check, diabetes mellitus, renal assessment, skin problem.

*Consider:*

- addressing the reminder to the pet;
- personalizing a pre-printed card by using the pets name;

- using humour to make it eye-catching so that it is not just thrown away: mailing it in an envelope may have the same effect;
- giving brief information outlining benefits of the particular service to owner and pet;
- including a simple questionnaire to encourage questions about pet health;
- requesting a urine sample as an introduction to a senior programme;
- including name, address, and phone number;
- giving a time for a pre-booked appointment to encourage the owner to phone and change it and thus making contact with the practice.

## Client information pack

*Function:* to give the new client, or new puppy/kitten owner an introductory pack of information about the practice consisting of several brochures that explains the services it offers, and how to care for their pet.
*Information to include:*

- practice brochure, or at least practice details (name, address, telephone number, opening times, payment method, etc.);
- caring for your pet (species specific);
- specific information on vaccination, worming, neutering, dental care, senior health, etc.;
- dietary recommendations;
- practice newsletter;
- recommended boarding kennels/catteries, grooming parlours, etc.

## Client registration form

*Function:* to gain information about a new client and their pets; to raise concepts of preventive health care to the owner from the first meeting.

The details you obtain from this form can simplify the assessment of your client base, help you identify services that are needed, help with target mailing, and so on.

The questionnaire should not be too long or complicated. The practice name and logo should feature prominently, it should be confidential, and it should finish with, 'Thank you for your co-operation'.

*Questions you may wish to include:*

- Name, address, telephone number, and contact number of owner.
- How did client hear of the practice, for example Yellow Pages, practice sign, client recommendation ('Who may we thank?').
- Name, age, species, breed of pet.
- Health status of pet: neutered, vaccinated, last wormed.
- Any known disease or allergy problems with pet.
- Is pet on any medication?
- Weight of pet.
- What is pet fed?
- Does pet have any behaviour problems?
- 'We believe preventing disease is as important as treating it. Which of the following preventive health programmes for your pet would you like to know more about?' List . . .
- Any other pets? List . . .

## ▬▬ Sympathy/birthday/thank you for the referral/welcome to the practice cards

*Function:* to convey a particular, personalized message from the staff of the veterinary practice to create the feeling that you really care about the pets and their owners.
   *Consider:*

- handwriting the owner's/pet's name and the appropriate message;
- using the personal signature of one or all of the members of the staff;
- addressing the birthday/welcome card to the pet;
- including a small gift, or discount voucher for a health care product from the practice.

## ▬▬ Clinical examination form

*Function:* to simplify and standardize history and record taking for the benefit of the practice, client and referring veterinary surgeon.
   Forms can be produced for:

- general health examinations;
- skin cases;
- senior health checks;
- dental examinations;

- ophthalmology;
- neurological assessments;
- gastrointestinal problems;
- cardiology, etc. . . .

The general health forms can be used on a daily basis to standardize clinical examinations. Copies of them can be given to owners upon completion as:

- proof of a thorough examination;
- opportunity to stress that certain problems were identified during the examination which may need further investigation.

The other forms are used for:

- referrals to other veterinary surgeons;
- guides for examinations of body systems, especially when the user is not doing these regularly.

The forms should include:

- practice name, address, telephone and fax numbers;
- practice logo;
- space for the client's and pet's details and relevant history;
- simple diagrams where appropriate;
- questions that work logically through a system;
- space to write comments, observations, etc.

If the client is personally taking the pet to a referring veterinary surgeon the practice can provide a simple, pre-printed map of the location.

## ■■■ Client questionnaires

*Function:* to gain information about the client's view of the practice with the aim to improve the practice to better suit the client's needs.

*Subjects for questionnaires:*

- service both in general and specifically;
- assessment of the newsletter;
- understanding of particular articles in the newsletter, etc.;
- how the clients first found the practice;
- monitoring the effect of changes made in the practice;
- interest in new services.

Questionnaires can be anonymous or signed, targeted or random. Properly designed and used they are probably the most effective way of finding out what your client really wants.

Use the information generated to:

- compare branches of your own practice;
- improve your services;
- make changes in the organization and running;
- identify what your clients really want.

Questionnaires can be:

- mailed out to clients;
- completed while waiting;
- included in a newsletter as the response element.

## ■■■ Business documents – stationery, invoices, health certificates, business cards, compliments slips, envelopes, etc.

*Function:* to transact written business.

All these documents should include the practice logo, name, address, fax and telephone numbers. Invoices can also have seasonal information about services available in the practice.

## ■■■ Posters

*Function:* to promote services and goods to clients within the practice using a simple but powerful image or message.

Posters can be home-made or supplied by companies. They must have high visual impact to be effective so should not include a lot of text. They should, of course, only be displayed if the products or sevices they advertise are recommended by the practice.

Subjects suitable for posters include:

- health programmes, for example dentistry, senior, puppy parties;
- 'behind the scenes' displays of the practice showing practice facilities;
- forthcoming events;
- to raise awareness of new diseases or epidemics, etc.

*Appendix 3*

# Conducting Market Surveys

> *Superior performance . . . (in client service) . . . – however you measure it – is a matter of meeting your customer's requirements. And you can't meet these requirements if you don't know what they are. Not what you think they are or what you want them to be, but what they really are. How do you learn what they are? Very simply, you ask your customers what they want, need and expect, in a variety of ways. Then listen and act.*
> Cannie and Caplin, *Keeping Customers for Life*, 1991

Market surveys can range from small, in-practice questionnaires to a full investigation of your current and possible market by outside experts. The basic questions you want answers to are:

- Why do your clients come to you?
- How do they value your services and products?
- What do they like and dislike about your practice?
- How do you compare to your competitors?
- What do you do that annoys, infuriates or really pleases them?

These can then be adapted for a focus subject (such as the need for an obesity clinic; better telephone service).

There are several types of client insight research of which the most commonly used are:

## Direct personal contact with clients

It is very easy to ignore or dismiss as unimportant what clients are saying to you in a practice situation, but by consciously listening to them and asking probing questions you can find out what they really want. Often it is quite different from their apparent reason for coming to the practice.

Random phoning of clients who have been into the practice in the last few weeks can also give information about their impressions and what they want from their practice.

## ■■■ Staff contact with customers

Staff who are trained to listen are invaluable at picking up information from clients. They not only have the most direct idea of what is going on, but they probably have excellent ideas of their own too. Clients often chat more freely to staff members, so encourage all staff to pay attention to what clients say – then be prepared to use this information to make changes in the practice.

## ■■■ Feedback

Feedback is a common form of formal client research. A typical example is the card found in hotel rooms with a number of questions pertaining to the service in the hotel. Feedback provides very useful information but there are several points to remember:

- Keep systems, for example questionnaires as short and simple as possible.
- Use behaviours that measure satisfaction, for example would the client recommend the practice to a friend? What is the level of satisfaction with waiting time for appointments on a 1–5 scale?
- Share results of feedback systems so that everyone in the practice knows what clients think – good or bad.
- Tell clients you value their opinion because you really want to do something about the level of service you offer them.

## ■■■ Client questionnaires

Simple and effective client questionnaires can easily be prepared in the practice as long as the following guidelines are used:

- Focus on one problem area at a time, for example reception service, post-operative release of pet, routine vaccination service.
- Keep questions short and simple.
- Use predominantly closed questions (requiring a yes/no answer), or ones that have graded answers (What do you think of . . . on a 1–5 scale?).

- Use some open questions to learn what people think is important.
- Avoid asking more than 5–6 questions to ensure co-operation.
- Explain what the questionnaire is for.
- Thank clients for their help.
- Keep clients informed about progress.

## *Example of a feedback questionnaire*

Here at Rosewood Veterinary Hospital we would like to improve our telephone service to you, our valued clients and patients. Please help us assess our current service by circling your answers to the following questions:

1. Do you have difficulty contacting the practice?

   *Yes/No*

2. When you last phoned the practice, how quickly was the telephone answered?

   *<3 rings     3–5 rings     >6 rings*

3. Was the person who answered

*Friendly and helpful?*          *Indifferent?*          *Not helpful?*

4. (a)  Were you kept waiting on hold?          *Yes/No*
   (b)  If 'yes', how long for?

   *< 1 minute     1–3 minutes     > 3 minutes*

5. What suggestions would you make to help us improve our telephone service?

A questionnaire like this would give information on how well the phone is answered, and whether you need more incoming lines (or staff to handle calls). Other specific questions could ask whether the client was phoned back in the promised time, whether they felt all their questions were answered, and for how long they thought their conversation lasted.

There is an advantage to using external organizations to do client surveys – answers are likely to be more honest. However, bad answers or complaints should not be received in a negative light: they provide an opportunity to improve the service to clients.

## ■■■ Evaluation

Research helps you evaluate your ongoing programmes by providing information for assessing your performance. This information can then be used to make decisions about working towards performance goals.

*For example, an airport opened information booths to help travellers with problems or questions. As these were not very successful they investigated further. Researchers found that most of the passengers were satisfied with the service they had received – but only 5% of all passengers had used the booths because* **the rest did not know where they were**. *Airport officials improved the visibility and advertising of the booths and more passengers were then aware of them and could use them.*

Sources for information are:

■ your clients;
■ non-clients because they are potential clients and can give you a different perspective on things than your present clients;
■ staff who are in constant touch with clients and are an excellent source of information.

Of course, ask comparable questions of each group.

*A thought in closing: The US Office of Consumer Affairs conducted exit surveys of 200 customers of a well-known Washington retailer. The choices were* **very satisfied, moderately satisfied, moderately dissatisifed** *and* **very dissatisfied**.

*Fifty-four per cent of the respondents said they were very satisfied ... But ... How many of the customers giving ... (the moderately satisfied response, not a bad rating) ... had a specific complaint about something that happened in the store? ... All of them. And how many of the 92 customers who were less than very satisfied ... complained to anyone in the store? Zero. Not one of them said anything. And why not, do you suppose?*

*When asked they said, because they expected mediocre service, because they didn't believe anything would be done if they had complained, and because the store's level of service was about the same as that of its competition.*

*In summary, if you're just content to retain market share . . . (these results) may be good enough – at least until your competition offers better service.*

Cannie and Caplin, *Keeping Customers for Life*, 1991

# References and Further Reading

Armstrong, M. (1990). *How To Be An Even Better Manager* (3rd edn). Kogan Page, London.

Blanchard, K., Carew, D. and Parisi-Carew, E. (1993). *The One Minute Manager Builds High Performing Teams*. Fontana, London.

Blanchard, K., Oncken, W. and Burrows, H. (1990). *The One Minute Manager Meets the Monkey*. Fontana (Harper Collins), Glasgow.

Bloom, M. (1994). Have you sorted out your contracts of employment? *Veterinary Business Journal* 3, 44–45.

Bone, D. (1988). *A Practical Guide to Effective Listening*. Kogan Page, London.

Bradford, D.L. and Cohen A.R. (1984). *Managing for Excellence*. John Wiley, New York.

Bradford, L.J. and Raines, C. (1992). *Twenty-something: Managing and Motivating Today's New Workforce*. MasterMedia, New York.

Bush, B.M. (1992). Obesity in small animals, its causes, diagnosis and treatment. *Veterinary Practice Clinical Review* 1 (6), 1–2,4,6–7.

BVA (1988). *BVA Guide to an Agreement Between Principals and Assistants*. BVA Publications, London.

Cannie, J.K. and Caplin, D. (1991). *Keeping Customers for Life*. Amacom, New York.

Catanzaro, T.E. (1991). Two outside forces that will change the way you practice. *Trends*, Oct/Nov, 26–28.

Covey, S.R. (1989). *The Seven Habits of Highly Effective People*. Fireside, New York.

Covey, S.R., (1992). *Principle-centered Leadership*. Simon & Schuster, London.

Denny, R. (1993). *Motivate to Win*. Kogan Page, London.

Desatnik, R. (1987). *Managing to Keep the Customer*. Jossey-Bass, San Francisco.

Dooley, D.R. (1992). Negativity gets you nowhere. *Veterinary Economics* **July**, 46–49.

Drucker, P.F. (1966). *The Effective Executive*. Harper & Row, New York.

Drucker, P.F. (1968). *The Practice of Management*. Pan Books, London.

Drucker, P.F. (1994). The theory of business. *Harvard Business Review*, Sept–Oct, 95–104.

Elkins, A.D. and Elkins, J.R. (1987). Professional burnout amongst US veterinarians: How serious a problem?. *Veterinary Medicine* **82**, 1245–1250.

Emily, P. and Penman, S. (1990). *Handbook of Small Animal Dentistry*. Pergamon Press, Oxford.

Geneen, H.S and Moscow, A. (1985). *Managing*. Granada, London.

Hackman, J.R. (1994). Commenting on *The team that wasn't*. *Harvard Business Review* Nov–Dec, 22–38.

Hackman, J.R. (1995). Can empowerment work at Sportsgear? *Harvard Business Review* Jan–Feb, 26–28.

Harvey-Jones, J. (1989). *Making it Happen*. Fontana Paperbacks, London.

Hayes, R. and Watts, R. (1986). *The Corporate Revolution*. Heinemann, London.

Hill, J. (1993). First years in practice: experiences of young graduates. *Veterinary Record* **132**, 521–522.

Hodgkins, E.M. (1990). Bringing wellness to companion animals. *Partners in Practice* **3** (3). PO Box 148, Topeka, Kansas.

Hunt, J. (1981). *Managing People at Work*. Pan Books, London.

Jevring, C. (1993). Do your support staff lay golden eggs? *In Practice* **15** (4), 198–201.

Jevring, C. (1994). Improving your telephone technique. *Veterinary Business Journal* **4**, 22–25.

Jevring, C. (1994). Expanding the role of the veterinary nurse. *In Practice* **16** (2), 101–104.

Kotler, P. and Bloom, P.N. (1984). *Marketing Professional Services*. Prentice-Hall, New Jersey.

Kotler, P. and Clarke, R. N. (1987). *Marketing for Health Care Organisations*. Prentice-Hall, New Jersey.

Kübler-Ross, E. (1970). *On Death and Dying*. London, Tavistock Publications Ltd. Republished (1993) Routledge, London.

*Legislation Affecting the Veterinary Profession in the United Kingdom*. Royal College of Veterinary Surgeons, 32, Belgrave Square, London SW1X 8QP.

Little, G. (1992). How to merchandise a practice. *Veterinary Practice* **July**, 8–10.

Little, G. (1992). What's wrong with selling? *In Practice* **January**.

Loder, M. (1985). *Feminine Leadership*. Times Books, New York.

Lofflin, J. (1992). Merchandising: it works for him. Does it work for you? *Veterinary Economics* **May**, 37–51.

Maister, D.H. (1982). A question of balance. In: *Professional Service Firm Management* (5th edn). Maisters Associates Inc., Boston.

Maister, D.H. (1984). Quality work doesn't mean quality service. In: *Professional Service Firm Management* (5th edn). Maisters Associates Inc., Boston.

Maister, D.H. (1986). The professional firm lifecycle. In: *Professional Service Firm Management* (5th edn). Maisters Associates Inc., Boston.

Maister, D.H. (1991). How managers add value. In: *Professional Service Firm Management* (5th edn). Maisters Associates Inc., Boston.

Maister, D.H. (1991). A service quality programme. In: *Professional Service Firm Management* (5th edn). Maisters Associates Inc., Boston.

Maister, D.H. (1991). Solving the underdelegation problem. In: *Professional Service Firm Management* (5th edn). Maisters Associates Inc., Boston.

Maister, D.H. (1993). The power of practice leadership. *In: Professional Service Firm Management* (5th edn). Maisters Associates Inc., Boston.

McCurnin, D.M. (1988). *Veterinary Practice Management*. J.B. Lippincott, Philadelphia.

Morgan, N.A. (1991). *Professional Services Marketing*. Butterworth-Heinemann, Oxford.

Oldcorn, R. (1989). *Management*. Macmillan, London.

Pease, A. (1984). *Body Language*. Sheldon Press, London.

Peters, T. (1989). *Thriving on Chaos*. Pan Books, London.

Peters, T.J. and Waterman, R.H. (1982). *In Search of Excellence*. Harper & Row, New York.

Pettit, T.H. (1994). *Hospital Administration for Veterinary Staff*. Am.Vet. Pub.Inc., California.

Pritchard, W.R. (1989). *Future Directions for Veterinary Medicine*, Pew National Veterinary Education Programme, North Carolina.

*Receptionists Rule OK* (1992). Proceedings of symposium, Hatfield, Herts.

*Royal College of Veterinary Surgeons Guide to Professional Conduct* (1993). RCVS, 32, Belgrave Square, London SW1X 8QP.

Sheridan, J. and McCafferty, O.E. (1993). *The Business of Veterinary Practice*. Pergamon Press, Oxford.

Swift, B. (1994). How to communicate with your employees. *Veterinary Business Journal* 3, 9–11.

Tannen, D. (1992). *You Just Don't Understand*. Virago Press, London.

Vivian, M. (1994). Tightening up on stock control. *In Practice* 16 (5), 282–285.

Women in the Professions (1990). Report by UK Interprofessional group, Working party on women's issues, June.

# Index